The Psychiatry of Adult Autism and Asperger Syndrome

The Psychiatry of Adult Autism and Asperger Syndrome
A practical guide

Traolach S. Brugha
Professor of Psychiatry, University of Leicester,
Consultant Psychiatrist, Leicestershire Partnership NHS Trust,
Leicester, UK

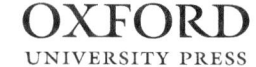

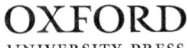

Great Clarendon Street, Oxford, OX2 6DP,
United Kingdom

Oxford University Press is a department of the University of Oxford.
It furthers the University's objective of excellence in research, scholarship,
and education by publishing worldwide. Oxford is a registered trade mark of
Oxford University Press in the UK and in certain other countries

© Traolach S. Brugha 2018

The moral rights of the author have been asserted

First Edition published in 2018

Impression: 1

All rights reserved. No part of this publication may be reproduced, stored in
a retrieval system, or transmitted, in any form or by any means, without the
prior permission in writing of Oxford University Press, or as expressly permitted
by law, by licence or under terms agreed with the appropriate reprographics
rights organization. Enquiries concerning reproduction outside the scope of the
above should be sent to the Rights Department, Oxford University Press, at the
address above

You must not circulate this work in any other form
and you must impose this same condition on any acquirer

Published in the United States of America by Oxford University Press
198 Madison Avenue, New York, NY 10016, United States of America

British Library Cataloguing in Publication Data
Data available

Library of Congress Control Number: 2017952751

ISBN 978-0-19-879634-3

Oxford University Press makes no representation, express or implied, that the
drug dosages in this book are correct. Readers must therefore always check
the product information and clinical procedures with the most up-to-date
published product information and data sheets provided by the manufacturers
and the most recent codes of conduct and safety regulations. The authors and
the publishers do not accept responsibility or legal liability for any errors in the
text or for the misuse or misapplication of material in this work. Except where
otherwise stated, drug dosages and recommendations are for the non-pregnant
adult who is not breast-feeding

Printed in Great Britain by
Ashford Colour Press Ltd, Gosport, Hampshire

Links to third party websites are provided by Oxford in good faith and
for information only. Oxford disclaims any responsibility for the materials
contained in any third party website referenced in this work.

Preface

Specialists in child psychiatry and in adult intellectual disability psychiatry can be expected to consider and diagnose autism. Within adult psychiatry, awareness of autism and the use of the terms 'Asperger syndrome', the 'autism spectrum' and 'high functioning autism', are growing in a few high-income countries, notably the UK and Sweden, and to some extent in the Netherlands, Australia, and North America.[1] However, autism has yet to become part of the accepted mainstream, core curriculum of adult psychiatry. In most of the world the term 'autism' still connotes a childhood condition, viewed as a subspecialty concern. There is a growing expectation, from outside of the profession, on psychiatrists to be able to recognize autism and consider its effects on their adult patients, particularly when they are also showing signs of another mental disorder, for example, psychosis, personality disorder or chronic depression. This expectation also extends increasingly to general practitioners and to clinical psychologists seeing adults.

Autism, including Asperger syndrome, was first described in children in the 1940s in Vienna and Baltimore (Silberman 2015). It has been shown since to be a strongly heritable condition. If suspected, autism can usually be diagnosed by the age of 2 or 3 years. The child fails to develop skills in reciprocal social interaction, understanding and flexibility, succinctly summed up in the phrase 'a failure to develop the social instinct'.[2] Because autism is significantly more common in the less intellectually able child, in the more able child it may be overlooked until adulthood. Epidemiological research has shown that most adults in the general population meeting criteria for autism are unrecognized and undiagnosed, and have unusually little contact with services.[3] Psychiatry could help to make autism more visible in

---

[1] Throughout this book, unless based on a cited source, such assertions represent the experience and opinion of the author.

[2] This apt phrase was communicated to the author by Dr Lorna Wing; it is not known who initially coined it.

[3] The author led the team that carried out this research throughout England.

adulthood, so that the health and mental health needs of those affected can be better addressed.

The aim of this book is to introduce autism[4] to psychiatrists[5] who see adults, including adult subspecialist psychiatrists, who are relatively unfamiliar with the topic. There is no book or similar source that the adult psychiatrist can turn to for a comprehensive introduction to autism and Asperger syndrome, written to fit with their perspective, and that caters to their learning and clinical practice needs. This book should assist them with its recognition and diagnosis in adulthood. It is designed to enhance their role in treating patients with co-morbid mental disorder, while understanding and taking account of the autism component. The purpose of this book is also to help in signposting patients with autism to appropriate care and support as family involvement diminishes or ceases in adulthood. It is hoped that it will also encourage psychiatrists in positions of influence to add their voice as advocates for people on the autism spectrum, which will help to bring about the new resources and care services required to support them. One day, it may help improve the lives of people with autism if hoped for developments in medical treatments emerge.

There are many books on autism in childhood, and on methods for supporting children and their families, mainly written by non-psychiatrists. There are a few books, including some by adult women and men with the condition, on how to cope with autism, including when family support has ended or is no longer appropriate. There are a number of academic monographs, usually multi-author, on autism research, mostly in childhood, with limited value for adulthood. There is no book on autism for the practicing adult psychiatrist comparable with the many textbooks available on the other major mental and behavioural disorders.

Teaching adult psychiatrists about autism has generated important experience of the busy psychiatrist's learning needs (learning needs will be reflected on in the final chapter). It has shown the considerable strengths psychiatrists bring to the subject, for example, experience and great skill

---

[4] The term 'autism' is used throughout this book. This is an abbreviation of 'autism spectrum disorder' (ASD) the current recommended name of the condition (DSM-5; American Psychiatric Association 2013). As explained in Chapter 1, these terms have now replaced the former official terms 'Asperger syndrome', 'high functioning autism' (HFA), 'childhood autism', and 'pervasive developmental disorder' (PDD). These changes are expected to be reflected in ICD-11 (forthcoming).

[5] This book should also be of value to the primary care physician and clinical psychologist already familiar with adult psychiatry, its terminologies, and its conventions.

in patient interviewing and direct observation, team work, managing the care and support of adults across a range of health and social care agencies, including specialist hospital units, housing, work, welfare, and adult education. It has also brought to light the challenges that many psychiatrists face in incorporating and integrating into their knowledge of adult mental and behavioural disorders an understanding of autism. It has shown how important it is for adult psychiatrists to gather and consider in sufficient detail information on early childhood development and current social development by interviewing informants such as parents and appropriate others in order to clearly differentiate lifelong neurodevelopmental impairments from conditions emerging late in childhood or in adult life.[6]

Given the educational and training needs of the profession, the approach taken here is similar to textbooks in other branches of medicine and psychiatry that describe normal and pathological functioning, and describe and guide the reader through assessment and post-diagnostic intervention issues. Use will be made of clinical vignettes that have been helpful in illustrating autism and its presentation in adulthood, which have worked effectively in training. These help to illustrate the issues psychiatrists raise in training workshops. The layout of the book is similar to that of a care pathway with chapters devoted to recognition, consideration of whether assessment for possible autism is warranted, followed by further steps towards increasingly detailed assessment and care planning.

In marked contrast to autism in childhood, there is an extremely limited published research literature and evidence base on autism in adulthood. Filling part of this gap are a small number of clinical and epidemiological research studies and systematic reviews, which will be cited and discussed. Therefore, in writing this book, I have had to rely heavily on my own clinical experiences and those shared with me by my professional peers. I acknowledge that there are risks in any attempt to fill in the gaps in the relatively little that we know about the subject. Differences of opinion are more likely where there are significant gaps in knowledge; not everyone may agree with the approach taken here. It might have been the easier route not to proceed. However, I have been encouraged by the large numbers of adults in the population whose difficulties on the autism spectrum are still largely

---

[6] As an adult general psychiatrist, the author has worked with child and adult learning disability psychiatrists, under the auspices of the Royal College of Psychiatrists (RCPsych, London), to provide brief introductory training courses on autism for adult general and subspecialist psychiatrists, throughout the British Isles. General practitioners and clinical psychologists have also taken part.

unrecognized, some of whom, together with their carers, have left a mark on me, over the past two decades.

In conclusion, this book is written for adult psychiatrists throughout the world, in training or in clinical practice, and for all physicians and clinical psychologists with an interest in and responsibility for adults with behavioural and mental disorders.

Acknowledgements

The author gratefully acknowledges the support, suggestions, and critical feedback of Dr Tom Berney, University of Newcastle; Dr Peter Carpenter, Bristol; Dr Ian Davidson, Cheshire and Wirral; and Mr Tony Davis and Mrs Maire Brugha, Leicestershire, England.

Contents

Part I **Introduction and Background**

1. History and development of the concept of autism *3*
2. Awareness of autism in adulthood *13*
3. Development of behaviour and functioning (with hindsight) *33*
4. Autism as a lived experience *61*

Part II **The Clinical Assessment and Diagnostic Pathway**

5. Obtaining an assessment *79*
6. Initial assessment ('Triage') *95*
7. Full assessment: the developmental history *113*
8. Full assessment: interviewing the patient and autistic phenomenology *127*
9. Full assessment: direct observation and the signs of autism *137*
10. Comorbidity assessment *153*
11. Detailed needs assessment *169*

Part III **Care and Intervention after Diagnosis**

12. Approaches to treatment and care *183*
13. Social care, the personal passport, and reasonable adjustments *195*
14. Caring communities and caring societies *207*
15. Choices in life, and the awareness, knowledge, and skills to support them *215*

Appendices

Appendix 1. Epidemiology methods *225*

Appendix 2. The author's experiences in epidemiology and in policy development *227*

Appendix 3. Development of a new approach to interviewing adults about their experiences of autism based on the Schedules for Clinical Assessment in Neuropsychiatry (Chapter 8) *231*

Appendix 4. Independent evaluation of the ADOS in community populations *235*

References *237*

Index *249*

Part I

Introduction and Background

Overview of this book: learning objectives

This book is set out in three parts, the first addressing background ('pre-clinical') knowledge, the second assessment skills, and the final part care and support. The busy reader is free to select any part they feel best serves their learning needs, at a particular time. Core features of autism will be mentioned within all three parts in their respective contexts. Therefore, the diligent reader who starts with Chapter 1 and progresses sequentially through the book, chapter by chapter, will encounter some repetitiousness that may irritate.[1]

Three learning perspectives will be used in Part I, in the next three chapters (Table 1.1). First (in Chapter 2), ways of increasing awareness of the possibility of autistic characteristics, or indeed of autism itself, in others including our patients will be set out. Second (in Chapter 3), variations from population developmental norms will be reviewed. Ideas of what may underpin autism will be followed by a consideration of variations in psychological development that point to the likelihood of a diagnosis.

---

[1] Others may appreciate that repetition is an age old effective learning strategy.

Table 1.1 Learning about autism in adulthood, perspectives, topics, and tasks

Chapter	Perspectives	Knowledge covered	Learning objectives
2	Our noticing and our overlooking autism	Awareness of autism in adulthood	Acting on alerting characteristics of autism
3	Parental account of atypical (abnormal) developmental signs in autism	Psychological development with the benefit of hindsight	Knowing and understanding developmental signs
4	Personal perspectives of adults with autism	Autism as a lived experience	Psychopathology and phenomenology of autism

Third (in Chapter 4), what people living with autism can tell us about their experiences and their perspectives will be used to expand knowledge of the subject.

In Part II of this book, the skills needed for assessment and for determining who would benefit from an assessment (Chapters 5 and 6) will be described. Assessment will be based on three complementary approaches:

- history of early psychological development and current functioning as viewed by carers (Chapter 7);
- information gained directly from interviewing the patient (Chapter 8);
- information based on direct observation (Chapter 9).

Assessment of comorbidity with other mental disorders (Chapter 10) and additional assessments in more severe cases of autism will be covered in Chapter 11.

In Part III approaches to care and support following diagnosis will be described that range from the traditional 1:1 perspective through the wider social care perspective, involving key others through to the public health, policy, planning, and evaluation perspectives.

Chapter 1

History and development of the concept of autism

Definition

Before describing some of the history of the development of autism as an idea and as a concept it is necessary to consider how it has been defined. Autism remained unclearly defined and, therefore, almost impossible to study empirically in its earliest years.[2] Individual researchers such as Gillberg (Gillberg and Gillberg 1989), and the World Health Organization and the American Psychiatric Association began to change that.

Autism is currently defined in the American Psychiatric Association fifth revision of the Diagnostic and Statistical Manual (DSM-5; American Psychiatric Association 2013) by the presence of two characteristics:

- persistent deficits in social communication and social interaction across multiple contexts;
- together with restricted, repetitive patterns of behaviour, interests, or activities.

It is a condition that emerges early in childhood, appearing to be far more common in males than in females, and which can lead to long-term social isolation and difficulties in fitting into school and employment settings throughout life. In later chapters in the first part of the book these features will be explored together with how to assess them in detail.

Although widely lauded, and the culmination of much work and international consultation, the DSM-5 definition, and the complete diagnostic criteria set out in the APA Manual, are best considered as work in progress. In particular, most of the authors are largely experts in understanding the condition in childhood. Although this revised definition makes clearer reference to the context of adulthood, there is less than one would wish to guide clinicians in adult practice, particularly in regard to the growing ageing population worldwide.

---

[2] Arguably, this was also true of other behavioural and mental disorders.

There is a growing expectation that the World Health Organization 11th revision of the International Classification of Diseases (ICD-11) criteria and clinical guidelines for autism, once finalized, will be similar to the DSM-5 definition. Ratification and publication are expected in 2018 following a period of field-trial studies by WHO.

Whether any of these behavioural and mental disorder concepts or constructs can be considered as disease entities (or medical conditions) in the way that better understood conditions in medicine are, such as diabetes, neuroblastoma, and hepatitis, is the subject of debate (Waterhouse et al. 2016). The disciplines of psychiatric epidemiology and psychiatric genetics are also taking an interest in empirically testing, such disease concepts. However, there is surprisingly little evidence of classifiers paying attention to such research when revising their official nomenclatures.

It is important and helpful to have some understanding of how the concept of autism developed over earlier years, in the very young history of the subject, for at least two reasons. First, this latest DSM definition is unlikely to be the final statement on the matter. Second, clinicians need to be aware of the current levels of uncertainty of the concept of autism (or of the autisms) and to act with appropriate flexibility in clinical practice in the light of this realization. This chapter aims to cover these issues applying them as far as possible to clinical experience of seeing how autism appears to affect younger and older adults.

History

The historical development of the concept of autism has been influenced by key historical figures, which is not terribly different, as psychiatrists know, from the development of other mental disorder diagnostic concepts. Two authors, neither of them professional historians, have provided informative and contrasting recent overviews of the history of the development of the concept of autism (Feinstein 2010; Silberman 2015). Feinstein, who is well known in the field of autism, a carer of an autistic child, interviewed many of autism's founding figures and quotes their words extensively. Silberman, a celebrated USA journalist, relatively new to autism, relied on secondary sources. Both authors addressed the curious issue that the concept was described in writing at approximately the same time by Kanner (1943) and by Asperger (1944). Both came from similar parts of central Europe and their respective first publications on the topic appeared during the same era, but on different continents.

Kanner had emigrated to the USA many years before his first publication on the subject. He had already achieved prominence as the author of the first major text book in child psychiatry, in which he showed no awareness of the concept. Kanner eventually rose to practice at the Harriet Lane Children's Hospital of John Hopkins University Medical School, Baltimore, and his first paper (in English), describing 11 children (Kanner, 1943), became widely regarded as the defining moment in the emergence of the concept of autism.

Asperger spent his career in German-speaking Europe and practiced in Vienna as a paediatrician, with an interest in children with brain damage and problems with learning for which they were provided with specialized training. Silberman's book emphasized the growing emergence over a decade or so of the concept of what we now call autism in Asperger's clinical practice, and in his teaching of many young doctors who trained with him in Vienna. (Kanner was not one of Asperger's trainees, but Silberman poses the question, unanswered so far, what did Kanner know or learn of Asperger's apparently long-incubating ideas?).

Asperger emphasized the strengths and sometimes exceptional skills of his patients. Silberman discusses the speculative idea that this might have been in order to try to protect them from Nazi eugenicists, who were literally exterminating intellectually disabled people including children. In contrast, Kanner emphasized the severity of the difficulties of his children and, it appears, regarded autism as a rare condition, diagnosing remarkably few cases in a long career in clinical practice. The word autism or autistic was coined by both Kanner and Asperger. Asperger published his paper in German in 1944. Lorna Wing was the first to bring to a wider readership attention to his paper (Wing 1981). It was subsequently translated into English and published in 1991 by Ute Frith (Asperger 1944, 1991).

The term Asperger syndrome became known after Asperger's death, possibly assisted by the widely read and influential article in *Psychological Medicine* by Dr Lorna Wing (Wing 1981).[3] Lorna Wing later shared with her colleagues some regrets about the 'success' of the term Asperger syndrome. She did not believe that there were two different kinds of autism (i.e. Kanner's and Asperger's), but rather that autism existed as a cluster of conditions that she termed a 'spectrum'.[4] Lorna's paper probably also served for the first time to bring the concept of autism out of its 'nursery' (childhood) in a journal read mainly by highly research active adult clinicians and their colleagues in psychology, epidemiology, and in the neurosciences.

---

[3] The author began to work with Lorna Wing at the MRC Social Psychiatry Research Unit in the year following Lorna's publication.

[4] The idea of autism as a continuous dimension came later.

Kanner's perspective on autism became widely known during the fifth, sixth, and seventh decades of the twentieth century. Therefore, it largely existed only in the world of child psychiatry and was very much driven by USA post-war developments in that discipline. This seems to have meant that only the most severe cases of autism were given the diagnosis—often these children were also affected by other forms of brain damage, including in particular intellectual disability, but sometimes also epilepsy. Regrettably, autism was also touched in the form of spurious and damaging ideas suggesting that it could be caused by maternal behaviour (in the form of psychological coldness or aloofness, as in the so called 'refrigerator mother'), which developed during the relatively short-lived period of dominance, by psychoanalytical ideas, of post-world war two USA psychiatry. The legacy of that period is that it has become more difficult, until now, to suggest ideas for research on how family functioning could influence early psychological development and outcome, in the context of families with a child with autism.

Asperger's concept, which embraced a wider range of general ability levels, only became fashionable from the 1980s onwards, which may explain several aspects of the development of the concept of autism that are still a problematic part of its historical legacy. First was the impression that Kanner and Asperger had discovered two different conditions, albeit related in some way. No accepted evidence of discontinuity of the statistical distribution of clinical features of children with these two diagnostic labels has been shown; a multisite study in the USA also showed complete inconsistency in the clinical use of these and other terms in children and young people (Lord et al. 2012). The fifth revision of the DSM took account of this realization in recommending abandonment of terms for subtypes of autism, including the term Asperger syndrome. This shift was much to the disappointment of many whose first diagnosis was given as Asperger syndrome by their doctor and who felt that, in some way, they were being cast back into the dark without a diagnosis.[5]

Splitting of the terms autism and Asperger syndrome seems to persist in the public mind.[6] Health service managers in the UK National Health Service (NHS) often use the term autism to apply to individuals with

---

[5] When communicating their diagnosis to a patient, the medical term 'autism' or 'autism spectrum disorder' may be preferable when seeking medical support. The words 'Asperger' or 'Aspie' may be more acceptable when a patient is talking informally to others about their condition.

[6] In public usage, the term autism seems to connote a severe disability of childhood. The term Asperger syndrome seems to suggest a high functioning teenager or exceptionally able adult.

co-existing intellectual disability, and use the term Asperger syndrome for individuals who are functioning at a higher level or independently as adults. These splits have various effects, some of them unhelpful (until recently, only the first of these two groups would have been allocated funding). They have made it difficult to ensure that services are developed in such a way as to address the distinct needs and preferences of all people with autism in accordance with their general ability and independence levels. The separation of services in this way (where any services exist) has also led to statistical reporting being separate. An anomaly of this is that the hugely influential Global Burden of Disease (GBD) Programme, until now, has reported separately childhood autism and Asperger syndrome statistics (Baxter et al. 2015). Therefore, studies that do not use these subtypes were not included in the GBD reports.

However, perhaps, the greatest problem of all with this separation and with the later emergence of Asperger's influence has been the broadening of the concept and the scope of autism. This seems to have brought with it greater recognition and more autism case diagnoses, but with the proliferation of the idea that the prevalence of the condition is rising in the population, i.e. that there is an epidemic of autism. Parallel influences have been the gradual acceptance that autism is not a binary condition (either present or absent), but exists on a continuum, ranging from the many individuals who have a few mild autistic traits through to the severely affected child or adult incapable of functioning safely without constant care and protection.

Before leaving the topic of perceptions of the concept of autism it is important to mention the helpful concept of neurodiversity (Lancet (Editorial) 2016). In general, diseases are thought of as disabling, unwanted, and unhealthy. Growing numbers of higher functioning individuals on the autism spectrum do not accept this view of their experience of living with autism. Instead, they prefer the idea of 'difference', rather than of 'disorder'. In support of this is the observation that people on the autism spectrum often have skills and abilities that stand out from their usual level of functioning, such as exceptional rote learning, recollection of detail, and logical reasoning. Higher rates of diagnosis have been reported in specific communities, such as in Silicon Valley, adjacent to major technological hubs, which may reflect that in technology and engineering populations and communities there may be more individuals with autistic traits that lend themselves to high levels of achievement in these employment settings. The idea of pride in autistic diversity is thus taking hold (Lancet (Editorial) 2016). This may help to reduce the stigma associated with autism, and it may also help people with the condition to fight successfully for their rights to full inclusion in society, including the right to work and live in the same community as others. This is an idea that will come up again in the last two chapters of this book on the development of autism-informed communities and societies.

Epidemiology

Classically, epidemiology has provided public health warnings to doctors to increase vigilance with regard to symptoms and clinical presentations that might otherwise go insufficiently recognized. Such information is also important for clinical practice in that epidemiology can identify differences between clinical expectation and actual findings in the wider population. Important questions of this kind about autism in adulthood are also beginning to be addressed by epidemiologists. They include the answer to how many people are affected by autism and how common it is in different adult age groups and according to gender. Governments, policy makers, and planners also need answers to these questions.[7] This need for policy information and how it is affecting service funding and developments for autism will be picked up in Chapter 14 of this book.

Detailed information on the methods used to obtain such information can be found in Appendix 1, Epidemiology methods. The key research findings and messages are summarized here.

In children, the median rate of autism for 16 surveys published in the period 1966–1991 was 4.4/10,000, whereas that for the 16 surveys published in the period 1992–2001 was 12.7/10,000. In three recent large region-wide or national surveys of children and young people in England, the prevalence of autism was approximately 10 per 1000 (Baird et al. 2006; Baron-Cohen et al. 2009; Green et al. 2005). It is agreed by most researchers that this reported increased prevalence is an artefact of case-finding differences and is unlikely to reflect any true increase in incidence due to newly emerging causes (Hill et al. 2016). Appendix 1, Epidemiology Methods, also summarizes surveillance work used to examine trends in diagnoses in the USA.

Findings of the first epidemiological study of autism in adults living in private households in England were published almost two decades following the above childhood studies (Brugha et al. 2009; Brugha et al. 2011). In England, rates of autism in adulthood show little significant evidence of decline with increasing age (Brugha et al 2009, 2011). Accordingly, policy on support for people with autism has been developed to cover all age groups, including over 65s (see Box 1.1) (Department of Health 2015). The importance of recognizing autism in older adulthood is beginning to receive more

---

[7] Economists point out that such information is needed in order to assist with the key question facing any country—what to spend money on.

Box 1.1 Example of statutory guidance on support for older adults in the light of evidence that autism also affects this older age group

Supporting older adults with autism

Older adults with autism are a neglected group and have received less attention through policy, research, and service provision. In part, this is because autism was only identified in the 1940s and the first generation of adults to be diagnosed are only now moving into older age. It is clear that approaches to older people with autism will need to change and develop.

The key message for local authorities and NHS bodies is that they need to plan appropriate services for older people with autism who live in the area, and ensure that mainstream services used by older people are appropriate for people with autism. Data collection is integral to the success of local planning, as will be incorporating this data in to local autism strategies and commissioning plans.

Local areas should have a diagnostic pathway in place for autism. They must ensure this works for older people, who report problems in being identified, not being able to provide a developmental history and additional health problems as obstacles to receiving a diagnosis.

Older adults with autism frequently rely solely on their families and friends for support. Preventative services will be particularly important for older adults with autism who are not eligible for social care support. Furthermore, special consideration is needed when planning for the transition into older age and the increased likelihood of other health issues, particularly when family may not be around to support adults with autism.

Source: data from Statutory guidance for Local Authorities and NHS organisations to support implementation of the Adult Autism Strategy, Copyright 2015, Department of Health attention from academic researchers, from people with autism, and from their carers (Wright 2016).

The most recent prevalence estimate, combining two adult household surveys in 2007 and 2014, is 7 cases per 1000, with a 95% confidence interval of 5–13 per 1000. This means that there is a 19 out of 20 chance that the true prevalence of autism in adults in England lies somewhere between these two estimates (between 5 and 13 per 1000). This estimate is within the range reported in the most recent childhood studies mentioned previously. These new adult surveys together also show that autism is far commoner in males than in females in the general population, as has been the case in the earlier studies of children. However, in adults with moderate to profound intellectual disability, there seems to be no sex difference in the prevalence of autism (Brugha et al. 2016). A final important finding for clinicians is that there is a significantly increased risk of epilepsy in adults with autism living in the community (Rai et al. 2012) whose autism, as already mentioned, is largely undetected and undiagnosed.

Associated factors in adulthood

Just as important as the prevalence of a condition are the factors that are associated with it, such as the characteristics of people with the condition found in the general population (which may differ from the types of people with the condition coming to the attention of services). In later chapters consideration will be given to these associations in the context of recognition, assessment, diagnosis, and care in adulthood. Among the clearest and the most important are the strong associations in adulthood with reduced verbal IQ and educational attainment, poorer living and social circumstances, social isolation, and under use of health care services (Brugha et al. 2011).

Strong associations with comorbidity include increased risk of adult attention deficit hyperactivity disorder (ADHD) in particular, but also a range of other mental disorders (see Chapter 10). There is also growing evidence suggesting increased risk of self-harm and suicide (Kato et al. 2013). Interest continues in the issue of possible reduced survival (increased mortality) in autism (Bilder et al. 2013; Hirvikoski et al. 2016).

Epidemiological methods also pave the way to the understanding of the genetic background to a condition, and to mapping its salient features and possible boundaries, with other disorders or conditions. Amongst the most important for clinical practice are two—the heritability of autism and the extent to which it is closely associated with comorbid conditions that it may even be confused with, masked by, or indeed, might mask and conceal (see Chapter 10).

The initial recognition and description of autism was soon followed by the frequent clinical observation of a strong family history of traits of autism in the family. This apparent association led to the development of the concept of the broader autism phenotype (BAP). Evidence for the strong heritability of autism was demonstrated in the first of several twin studies, based on collections of twins seen and diagnosed at autism clinics. It was recognized that findings based only on people identified through specialist clinics might not represent the wider population of people with autism and traits of autism in the general population, many of whom do not receive a diagnosis. One way of resolving this came about through the development of a major population twin register in the United Kingdom, based on twins, identified through sources such as birth registers, independently of the presence of any medical or behavioural condition (Colvert et al. 2015).

This work showed that liability to autism specifically, and importantly to a broadly defined index of traits of autism, was accounted for mainly by additive genetic effects (the addition of genetic and environmental effects). Environmental effects that are not shared (i.e. occurring outside the family) played a lesser, but nevertheless, significant role in heritability. Results were largely consistent across different methods for measuring the presence of autism. There was also considerable overlap between genetic factors that explain individual differences in traits that are autism-like and in the diagnosis of autism.

One might ask how specific are these findings to autism, as compared with other conditions? Epidemiology, when combined with genetic research methods, can also help inform us as to whether what we think of as a specific condition, or disorder, is actually just part of a larger group of seemingly similar or related behavioural problems. Might they reflect influences on a broad range of factors that influence the development of the brain, of social understanding and behaviour, including modes of communication that go beyond autism? A thought-provoking review of these problems has been published recently (Waterhouse et al. 2016).

A second study, based on the same UK population twin series, examined this question further (O'Nions et al. 2015), comparing genetic liability in children with autism with children with callous unemotional traits, asking the question are they separate or part of a single larger problem? The result was that genetic and environmental influences on these two sets of characteristics, autistic traits and callous unemotional traits, were quite distinctive. Further such studies can be expected to follow.

Currently, it is realized that underlying this inheritance is a far more complex, but possibly less clinically useful picture. Most cases are sporadic leaving no simple Mendelian pattern here upon which to base genetic counselling. Instead *de novo* mutations, micro-DNA deletions, and duplications are frequently encountered, and each family seems to be different to the next.[8] Clinicians working in this area come across multiply affected families where siblings who are not autistic are the exception. Environmental and epigenetic factors also seem to be at play.

Within the broader field of adult mental and behavioural disorder, various statistical classification methods, including mathematical taxonomic methods, have been used to test clinical theories of different types and subtypes of mental disorders. To date, these methods have not yet been used with adult data to study autism and to study potentially related behavioural syndromes. As mentioned earlier, classification methods have been used across different clinical sites showing that there was no consistent use of terms denoting subtypes of autism including Asperger syndrome (Lord et al. 2012). However, it is possible that if and when such studies are carried out, autism (or the 'autisms') will stand out clearly from other forms of mental and behavioural disorders.

Other factors shown to be associated with autism, in children identified through the services, include maternal polycystic ovary syndrome, pre-eclampsia, maternal infection during pregnancy, maternal gestational diabetes, neonatal birth weight or gestational age abnormalities, neonatal Apgar score, and parents with high abilities in mathematics and engineering (Modabbernia, et al, 2017).

The studies described in this chapter also show how important it is to adopt a quantitative, dimensional approach, as well as a binary (present versus absent) approach to identifying cases of autism. This will have implications for recognition, assessment, and management topics to be considered in the chapters to follow.

---

[8] However, mapping of rare genes to populations may help and support affected families by introducing them to other families that share the same extremely rare forms of abnormal development.

Chapter 2

Awareness of autism in adulthood

Background

Until recently, most assessments for autism were being conducted during childhood only. The necessary information was immediately available from parents (or equivalent guardians) and teachers. The child could be observed directly in play and while with peers. The possibility of autism may need to be considered in an adult who has not already been assessed as a child. Information on childhood development is correctly regarded as fundamentally important in deciding if an individual has autism.

It has only recently been shown that autism is similarly prevalent in adult and old age as in childhood (Brugha et al. 2011). As most people alive now are adults this means that most people needing to be assessed for autism are adults. For older adults there is little or no prospect of information on early development being obtained from a surviving informant. Their parents, if alive, may not be able to recall their child's development in sufficient detail. The adult may have lost contact or may refuse to involve his or her family (this is not unusual in practice).

In later chapters approaches to assessment in the older adult, in the absence of reliable information on early development, will be covered—including consideration of other conditions in adulthood that may mimic autism, but may actually be a different problem.

Raising awareness

The first step in adult practice is creating awareness of when autism needs to be considered as a possibility. Severe cases of autism (and particularly if complicated by common co-morbidities such as intellectual disability and epilepsy) are more likely to be picked up before adulthood. Therefore, one is considering here the much commoner situation where, for whatever reason, autism was not given formal consideration in childhood and the person of concern now has to manage independently as an adult. Now that it is realized that autism in adulthood is being missed careful consideration needs to be given to what the possible clues are for autism.

There will be people known to many practitioners who may have at least some features or some 'traits' of autism. Until now it has not occurred to them to consider these persons in this way. In this chapter, possible pointers to autism will be reviewed—listing possible alerting characteristics. This will be followed by a series of self-reflective exercises to encourage the reader to think who they know already, who might display more subtle features of the condition, which they might not have considered in this way previously. Following on that, a series of more conspicuous case studies will be set out highlighting which aspects might be due to autism.

Where autism diagnostic criteria are not fully met it is important to consider the significance of those 'subthreshold' symptoms that are present. If it is diagnosed, level of severity is also important from mild to severe. In the previous chapter it was noted that this quantitative trait approach is being tested out in research on the heritability of autism. This has shown that quantitative traits that are widespread in the community are genetically influenced in the same way as is the formal diagnosis of autism, as binary outcome.

Awareness (of possible autism) calls for flexibility. To learn to be aware of and to consider the possibility of autism in a person or patient, one needs to reach beyond binary perception. So also when responding to concerns expressed to us by a carer, colleague, or anyone else who knows the person. Many of the parents of adults, who are now being assessed with autism, were seen in the past by respected professionals who did not accept the observations and concerns expressed about their child by its parents. This observation is also supported by a recent study[1] of random samples of adult patients, in contact with mental health services, where only about 1 in 5 cases of autism had come to the attention of their mental health team (approximately 1 in 20 of all cases under their care (Tyrer et al. 2013)). This underscores clearly the need for greater awareness of the possibility of autism in any adult psychiatry caseload. Similar findings of under recognition of autism in psychiatric practice have been reported in Sweden (Nylander and Gillberg 2001).

It can be argued that to be clinically effective (i.e. sensitive or even suspicious) it is actually necessary to spend a little time thinking about the value of grey (non-binary) over black and white (binary) thinking. Over the years,

---

[1] This refers to research due to be submitted for publication, funded by the NIHR CLAHRC programme, which included data collection in Leicestershire and Northamptonshire, England.

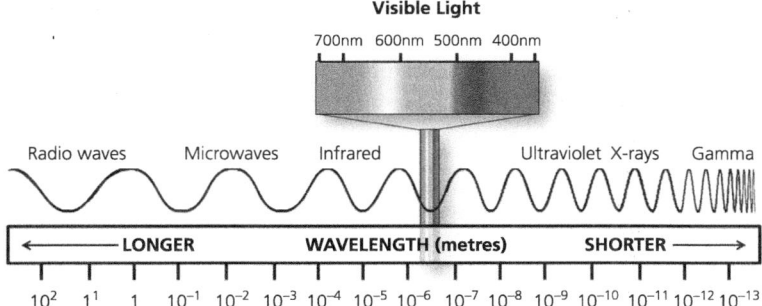

Fig. 2.1 The rainbow as a metaphor for our perception of distinct categories in a background of unbroken continuous change in the frequency of electromagnetic radiation.
Reproduced with permission from Florida Atlantic University.

conversations with people, including highly educated people, professionals, policy-makers, and journalists, re-enforce the unquestioned assumption that, in some sense, a patient either has or does not have a particular condition, be it medical, mental health (psychiatric), or autism. It would seem that we are designed to look at and quickly divide any behaviour we observe into 'normal' or 'disordered', and act upon that binary decision. Therefore, when we see puzzling or odd behaviour we are, as it were, forced into a rapid decision, to decide between 'eccentric but essentially normal', or clearly 'abnormal', 'disturbed', etc.

The rainbow metaphor is a useful way of pointing out how wrong (although evolutionarily successful) our thinking and perceptual process can be. What we perceive as the different colours of the rainbow, with seemingly clear lines of demarcation from one colour to the next, suggesting stark underlying differences, is mere illusion. At the level of the electromagnetic spectrum,[2] underlying the colours we perceive are smooth incremental increases (and decreases) in the frequency of the electromagnetic spectrum in the region we know as the visible light spectrum (see Fig. 2.1).

Why is this important—after all readers will already know this? Some readers may be surprised by the following assertion: you may never have considered or diagnosed autism, but it is suggested that you do already see it and know it around you, but perhaps you have never *thought of it in that*

---

[2] The electromagnetic spectrum is the collective term for the known frequencies and their linked wave lengths of electromagnetic radiation. The invisible components include radio waves, X-rays, infrared radiation and so on.

way. To develop skill and competency in diagnosing autism it is now being suggested that one can and needs to start with what we already know—even though we may not realize that one knows it.

Learning exercise

While training doctors about autism, they are asked to work for 5 minutes in pairs. Each participant is asked to think of someone they know as a person (not a patient or a colleague), who seems to fit with some of the descriptions of autistic traits observed in adults (Table 4.1), and to describe that selected person briefly to their fellow course participant. This can lead on to a lively and illuminating discussion of particular individuals and the difficulties they face in their lives. Rarely does any participant struggle to come up with a short or limited account of such a person. Experience with other groups of learners suggests that adult psychiatrists, although they may have little background in autism, but who choose to attend such training, perform well at this exercise.

What are the *alerting characteristics* that act as pointers to possible autism in an adult? Box 2.1 provides a list of alerting characteristics. These may look like diagnostic criteria and to some extent they are (see later chapters on assessment). For the purposes of this exercise it is suggested that each of the characteristics or traits in this table, can be seen from time to time in people we already know or, indeed, even in ourselves.[3]

The reader is encouraged to try the exercise for themselves. Read through the list in Box 2.1 and ask yourself who do you know that this reminds you of? Make a note of it.

Most people have one or several characteristics—only exceptionally socially able and often charismatic people do not seem to have any such characteristics at all. Having read through the list, are you reminded of anyone?

Try making notes:

- If you are thinking of a person with quite a lot of these characteristics ask yourself what has their life been like until now?
- Do they fit into the society around them like most people?

---

[3] There is, in the UK, the beginnings of recognition that doctors themselves may have concerns about having autistic traits and the need to be able to turn to someone with whom they can discuss this, not unlike the general issue of doctors with common mental health problems, such as depression, addiction, etc.

Box 2.1 Possible alerting characteristics of autism in adulthood

Autism presents in complex and varied ways. The following signs should encourage the clinician think of its possibility:

- Difficulties with social relationships (i.e. social isolation):
    - few or no sustained relationships—those that exist are likely to be either distant or intense;
    - persistent aloofness or awkward interaction with peers (which sometimes may be unduly compliant or passive);
    - unusually egocentric with little concern for others or awareness of their viewpoint, and limited empathy or sensitivity even with others described as friends;
    - lack of awareness of social rules—prone to social blunders.
- Problems in communication:
    - odd voice, monotonous, and perhaps at an unusual volume (too quiet or loud for the setting);
    - talking at (rather than to) you with little display of awareness of your response;
    - language is superficially good, but too formal, stilted or pedantic, and with difficulty in catching any meaning other than the literal;
    - rather wooden, impassive appearance with few gestures and a rather odd, poorly coordinated gaze that may either avoid looking directly at you or else look through you, and can be misinterpreted as furtive or aggressive, respectively (i.e. limited non-verbal communicative behaviour);
    - awkward or odd posture and body language.
- Absorbing and narrow interests, and the avoidance of change:
    - unrelentingly pursued interests;
    - unusually circumscribed interests that contribute little to a wider life (for example, collecting facts and objects that have limited practical or social value);
    - a set approach to everyday life that may include unusual routines or rituals; change is often upsetting;

- unusual sensory differences, with over or under sensitivity to specific sounds, pain, heat or cold, texture (especially in food or fabric), or artificial light.
- Although its presentation may change and moderate with age, it has a childhood onset and is lifelong.

The great variation in form and intensity means that stereotypes can be misleading. In particular, as the presentation can be obscured by developmental change and successful compensation for disabilities, autism may only be revealed by the early developmental history.

Source: data from: Berney et al., CR136. Psychiatric services for adolescents and adults with Asperger syndrome and other autistic-spectrum disorders. Copyright 2006, Royal College of Psychiatrists.

- Do they seem to need help in managing common sense issues, including risks?
- Are they managing to live independently or still living with family?
- Is there something they rely on others to do for them to keep on going—or to keep safe?
- Do they realize how they seem or appear to others?
- What might be the effect of having this pointed out—or, indeed, what was the effect if this happened?
- Does it trouble them or are they essentially content if also dependent on one or more others?
- Do they have any strengths or particular skills? Do others find them useful, for example, when it comes to fixing things such as computer equipment or machinery when it does not seem to work?
- Are they chatty or very economical, only talking when spoken to and replying strictly to the point—or to the point as they see it?
- Or are they not dependent on others?
- Have they been able, or unable, to come through the inevitable ups and downs that life throws at most of us sooner or later? Or have they had surprisingly great difficulty?

If autism is a possibility, all of these questions will come into play in determining whether the benefits of considering that possibility further outweigh any possible disadvantages. This will be considered further in Chapter 5, on seeking an assessment.

> **Box 2.2 Factors associated with autism in adults in the general population**
> - Less likely to be in a long-term relationship, partnership, or marriage.
> - More likely to be living in rented accommodation.
> - Less well educated and having a lower verbal IQ.
> - More likely to be male.
> - More likely to be living in a deprived neighbourhood.

Unless we are open to the possibility of a broader spectrum of autism, ranging from mild and harmless eccentricity through to extremely impaired functioning, we may fail to consider the possibility of identifying and opening up options for support to someone who may be leading a difficult life, possibly as a result of autism. In the first adult general population survey (Brugha et al. 2011) a number of characteristics and possible consequences of autism were found, all of them in persons meeting assessment criteria for autism, but unrecognized, undiagnosed, and living in the community (Box 2.2).

These characteristics suggest that life is difficult if you have autism and live in the community, with your behaviours not understood as being due to a recognizable medical condition, for which you are not in any way responsible.

Case studies and case vignettes

In the next chapter the reader is invited to look at some examples of what having autism is like, from the perspective of the person with the condition. Before that it will be helpful to focus on signals and signs we may spot in our patients. Therefore, in this chapter the reader will now be encouraged to look at a series of individual personal accounts—of case vignettes—any of which could be a possible case of autism (and/or of another medical or psychiatric condition). There are seven such cases included here, which may seem daunting to the busy reader, but nevertheless, it is suggested that it would be well worth working through the first two or three, at least, before moving on to the next chapter.

In each case there will be several questions to consider. It is important to focus particularly on two:

1. What in the account is suggestive of the possibility of autism?
2. What else might underlie or explain the account?

To get the best out of what follows it is recommend that the reader try out these exercises themselves:

1. Make notes in response to the questions and instructions following each account.
2. Each will then be followed by a discussion of possible responses to the questions.
3. See how well you have done—how many had you thought of? (Every time these are used in training, something new and original does seem to come up).

Most are in the form of the familiar request for advice from a primary care-based family physician (general practitioner). We will begin by considering the above two questions in relation to each case study. First, from the information provided, what led you to consider an autistic spectrum disorder? Second, what other explanations for this account are there (most readers will find this important question the more straightforward of the two).

Case Study A

A referral to an adult mental health service from a primary care physician (i.e. a 'GP'):

> Dear Team
>
> I would be grateful for your advice on this 18-year-old young man who has hardly stepped out of the house since finishing at school last summer. His parents are distraught. He spends most of his time in his room watching television, videos, playing computer games, or online. Apparently he plays the same videos over and over again, seemingly quite contentedly.
>
> He has never had a girlfriend. He only sees his school friends about once a month and that is at the pub. The family say you can set your watch by the time he returns because it never varies. However, one night he did not come home until 2 a.m. when one of his friends left him at the front door. The next day when asked why he was so late he said 'this one "pulled me"[4]—she just wanted hot sex—she let me borrow the new Manga game for the PS2—wicked! …'. The parents could get no more information out of him.
>
> Occasionally, he gets frustrated and angry, usually with his mother, for example, if there is no Coca-Cola left in the house. He almost hit her once. The

---

[4] A phrase used in some cultures to denote being approached in a social setting, such as a party or a bar, by a person with a view to making personal contact that could develop into a sexual encounter.

parents occasionally hear him shouting in his room. His father has taken to staying out late. When I visited the home (he would not come to my surgery) he hardly responded to my questions, but told me that everything was fine. It was as if I wasn't even there. He did not show obvious signs of anxiety and depression.

There is a younger child in the house aged 12 who has told her mother that she is frightened and refuses to be left alone in the house with her brother. I appreciate that you may receive requests like this from time to time, but my reason for seeking advice is that the family situation seems increasingly concerning, and I do not know where else to turn for advice.

Now make some notes in response to the following questions.

1. The young man does not have a diagnosis, but from the information provided what would make you consider an Autistic Spectrum Disorder? (Underline the relevant parts of the account).
2. What other kinds of explanations could there be for this behaviour? (Other conditions apart from autism?)

List possible responses, and what each means or could mean, focusing on questions 1 and 2 above. (Do make a few notes before reading this—you will learn far more by trying—the 'more mistakes you make the more you will learn!')

Q1. He spends most of his time in his room watching television, videos, or playing computer games or online. Apparently, he plays the same videos over and over again seemingly quite contentedly. This suggests a preference for solitariness, routine, resistance to change, and possibly repetitive behaviour.

He has never had a girlfriend. He only sees his school friends about once a month and that is at the pub. This suggests he has great difficulty in making and, importantly in sustaining, friendships (there is repetitiveness, inflexibility in the pattern of contact, which is also infrequent).

Other pointers to possible autism are his brief outbursts of anger (emotional expression in autism even in adulthood appears to be underdeveloped and more like that of a young child), his vulnerability to sexual exploitation, and his lack of appreciation of potential risks.

Q2. Other possible explanations, other than autism, could be obsessive compulsive disorder, mild intellectual impairment, depression, anxiety, post-traumatic stress disorder, insidious onset of psychosis, the use of alcohol or drugs. The fact that he is content would argue against his repetitive behaviour being 'against conscious resistance', as in obsessive compulsive disorder. His anger could be part of a range of mental disorders—there is no other striking expression of emotion. He goes out drinking once per month, which could provide an opportunity to source other substances. Alcohol could also be used to reduce anxiety associated with social contact.

Case Study B

A known long-term patient with a new community mental health nurse (CMHN). He has been living alone for 4 years.

John is now aged 32 and seems very solitary. He has had one mental health acute admission—this was 4 years ago and followed a few weeks after his sole carer, his mother, died. According to the GP, he was then withdrawn and losing weight, and neighbours were complaining that his rubbish bin was overflowing and was not being taken to the street for collection day.

On admission for an assessment under the Mental Health Act, it was difficult to obtain a coherent account from him. He was withdrawn and avoiding other patients and staff. He was observed by night staff to be behaving as if he was hearing voices, which he did not acknowledge, when asked. When asked about this by the psychiatrist, he said that people were always looking at him and commenting on him in the street. He found it easiest to keep to himself.

One of his sisters visited him on the ward and brought in a collection of jigsaw puzzles that he soon became totally absorbed in. Cleaning staff tried to move one of the puzzles, which was on a table by his bed: when he saw what had happened he started screaming, and frantically waving his hands and arms. Several nurses came rushing to the scene, but they did not have to apply any physical restraints as he immediately cowered in a corner.

He was commenced on olanzapine, and seemed to become more relaxed and willing to sit in the day room watching TV with other patients. He never joined in the chit chat. No matter who was there he always switched on the evening news without asking if anyone minded—the other patients seemed to know that it was unwise to object.

Four years later he is still being seen at exactly the same time and day every 4 weeks by his CMHN. He also has support workers who help him keep the house tidy, check that he pays his bills on time, and go shopping with him to the local food store. He is still on the same medication, at a high dose, set on discharge, and is seen in the outpatient clinic by a trainee psychiatrist every 3 months. When asked about psychotic symptoms he replies 'oh that question again—no'.

1. What would make you consider an Autistic Spectrum Disorder? (Underline the relevant parts of the account).
2. What other kinds of explanations could there be for his initial presentation?

Discussion of questions 1 and 2. (Remember to make a few notes before working through this.)

Q1. The fact that he is avoiding other patients and staff, and that he soon became totally absorbed in jigsaw puzzles, is consistent with possible autism. His reaction, when staff tried to move one of the puzzles on a table by his bed, screaming and frantically waving his hands and arms, are consistent with an intolerance to change in one's surroundings, found in autism. Routines and resistance to change are seen in the observation that he preferred being seen at exactly the same time and day, every 4 weeks, by his community nurse, and by the observation in hospital that he always switched on the evening news without asking if anyone minded—the other patients seemed to know that it was unwise to object (possibly because of his reaction). The fact that he never joined in the chit chat, suggests difficulties in engaging in reciprocal social interaction. Needing continuing help to keep the house tidy and checking that he pays his bills on time are consistent with autism, even in someone with relatively high general ability. Such patients are potentially at considerable risk from neglect of their physical health—we should not presume that they are receiving attentive general health care locally.

Q2. Being observed by night staff to be behaving as if he was hearing voices is consistent with the original diagnosis of psychosis being correct. Indeed, he could have both autism and psychosis. Avoidance of others and the observation that, on the antipsychotic medication olanzapine, he seemed to become more relaxed and willing to sit in the day room watching TV with other patients could suggest social anxiety. The observation that there continue to be support workers who help him keep the house tidy, check that he pays his bills on time, and go shopping with him to the local supermarket could fit with mild intellectual disability.

Case Study C

A young woman was arrested for stalking a former teacher and released after being charged. She is reported to the police to be repeating her behaviour contrary to an order by a court and has been taken back into custody. The Police Surgeon has requested an appropriate adult due to her 'bizarre behaviour' and has requested advice from your team (this could be either a community mental health team or a local social care team).

The woman has been receiving a service from the Child and Adolescent Mental Health Services, but no diagnosis has been recorded. A recent transfer to the Local Adult Mental Health Team has been made. The woman's solicitor has also requested a report for court. It is alleged that she repeatedly writes letters, makes telephone calls, sends emails, and stands outside the home and or workplace of the teacher, waiting for her to leave or to return. The teacher is now on treatment from her primary care physician for stress.

The woman is described as dressing in an old fashioned style (she is now aged 18) and wearing very colourful make-up carelessly applied. She occasionally uses highly sexualized language at interview, although her expression does not indicate that she expects you to be shocked in any way by this. She does not seem to understand why there is a problem with her behaviour. She seems distracted, looking around the room and staring at details such as the window, door handle, electric wiring. When asked questions she seems to stare blankly at the questioner and if she replies, may often produce an irrelevant or inconsequential reply. It is difficult to get her attention.

1. What if any elements of this account would point to a possible case of autism (underline any phrases that suggest this)?
2. Although she does not have a diagnosis you may suspect an autistic spectrum disorder. From the information you have what would make you consider this? (Underline the relevant parts of the account.)

Discussion of questions 1 and 2.

Q1. Repetitive behaviour that is not easily altered by the expressed disapproval of others and particularly behaviour that is socially discouraged (repeatedly standing outside the teacher's home) should raise the possibility of autism. Not all cases of stalking are due to autism—it is important to consider autism, but also to accept that such behaviour may exist on its own in the absence of additional evidence of a more profound developmental problem. People with autism often dress in public in a way that does not fit in socially. We sometimes see in women with autism an attempt to mimic the appearance and dress of an idol with whom they are fascinated—this might be a celebrity or even a historic figure. Discussing openly and publically matters that most adults would regard as private may indicate a lack of understanding of social norms. Staring at physical objects (and possibly failing to use eye gaze directed at the person speaking to them) may also indicate attention to detail in autism and difficulties with non-verbal aspects of social communication. Replies to questions might seem quite out of context. From the perspective of the person with autism their reply might be highly logical, but over-literal, focusing on some detail that was not intended by the person communicating with them. A classic example is, when asked 'do you hear any voices when there is no one there,' to reply saying yes (referring to actually heard voices, but of persons in another room overheard).

Q2. Clearly, we would want to rule out the onset of psychosis or of an organically or drug-induced altered mental state including, very importantly, an acute confusional state. Staring at physical objects (perhaps 'distractedly') might suggest that the person is experiencing visual or auditory hallucinations. Such states are more likely to have a defined point or period of onset preceded by behaviour that is largely viewed as normal, whereas the difficulties in autism are lifelong. Repetitive behaviour might suggest an obsessional phenomenon; at interview it is important to differentiate behaviour carried out against conscious resistance ('compulsively'), and behaviour that the person chooses to repeat and if anything only gives rise to distress if prevented or inhibited by the action of others. Misunderstanding or seemingly not 'getting the point' of what is being said in an interview might suggest a mild intellectual disability.

Case Study D

Mr Fern lives in the community on his own in a three-bedroom house. He has a history of repeat offending behaviour, namely holding a knife while shouting at his neighbours, walking around with no clothes on, and masturbating in public toilets. He has had continuous difficulty living in close proximity with neighbours. Neighbours often complain that they can hear him shouting on the phone, talking to himself, and staring at people/into their windows from his back garden, late at night.

When questioned about his behaviour Mr Fern cannot understand how his behaviour makes other people feel or how they may be interpreted as socially inappropriate. Mr Fern finds it hard to finish conversations. He will repeat what he has said, often talking over other people, and does not recognize any prompts that the listener is not interested or needs to leave, unless it is spelled out to him, i.e. 'I'm going now'. He will also put the phone down if you say this when you are about to pass the phone to someone else.

When talking to him he often takes things very literally, e.g. when told 'I can't come, I'm snowed under', he commented, it wasn't snowing where he was (5 minutes away).

He often avoids places and people he is unfamiliar with and new activities. To those he knows well, he admits it is because he does not understand what they are saying to him or how he should behave. He has told people that he finds words with pictures next to them easier to understand.

Mr Fern often tells people things that seem not very nice, such as 'you look ugly on that photograph' or 'I don't like your new spectacles'.

He gets on well with rules; for example, he has been asked not to swear in front of particular people and to take turns in talking. However, he does not generalize these to other people or places, and has to have them set again. He can also interpret rules very concretely potentially putting himself at risk from others' reactions to him. For example, if he notices someone swearing in public he may publically criticize them.

1. What are Mr Trimble's difficulties which might point to autism (e.g. problems in imagination, communication, social skills)?
2. What other kinds of health and mental health difficulties might this account suggest?

Discussion of possible responses and what each means or could mean.

Q1. Most of the behaviours listed point specifically to some aspect of autism, in particular, difficulties in relating to other people and knowing how to moderate his own behaviour. Offensive behaviour, and shouting or talking loudly in close proximity to others are apparent. He is unable to recognize the effect his behaviour has on others, although the reactions of others may make that clear. His difficulty in learning from his errors and his lack of grasp of the level of offence his behaviour can cause others stands out. There is also a rigidity and inflexibility about his behaviour, and a proneness to repeat the same behaviours.

Q2. Mr Fern also shows some signs of possibly having a degree of intellectual disability. This should be considered further. His overall level of activity would suggest that he is now slowed down or depressed (or, indeed, elated), and also that if he has anxiety symptoms they are not obvious. Some of his behaviour in public might raise other concerns that should also be considered—shouting at his neighbours, walking around naked in public, and masturbating in public areas. Before asking an autism or intellectual disability team to consider working with him, the possibility of an unrecognized psychosis should be ruled out by a doctor or mental health-qualified professional. His physical health should also be monitored as he may not be able to take responsibility for this.

Case Study E

Mrs Smith calls the local social care Duty Team with concerns for her neighbour Peter, aged 35, who lives next door to her. He had been found 'loitering' around the chip shop on Friday night, looking surprisingly dishevelled (wearing dirty clothes, which Mrs Smith had never seen before). He had got upset and agitated when the shop assistant wouldn't give him his fish and chips because he didn't have enough money. Mrs Smith said she paid for the fish and chips and this seemed to calm him down. He went home with two portions of fish and chips, but without even thanking her.

The neighbour reported that Peter had been living alone for a couple of weeks since his mother was taken into hospital. Peter's mother had left just enough money for Peter to get his share of food. Mrs Smith described Peter as a quiet man mostly, apart from a few times, 'like in the chip shop, when he gets upset'. Mrs Smith stated she had attempted to help Peter by bringing him some dinners, but he had not always eaten them and the plates are starting to pile up unwashed. Although she had heard the vacuum cleaner, Mrs Smith suspected he spent most of his time in his room, possibly in his bed. She had not seen Peter leave the house since his mother went into hospital, apart from the incident at the fish and chip shop, and as far as she was aware he didn't go to work.

According to Mrs Smith, Peter's mother had told her that Peter needed a lot of help with taking care of himself. He seemed ok to her and would be seen to help his mother a lot, which was a shame because he didn't really get a chance to have a life of his own. As far as she was aware he had never left home and she had not noticed any friends come to visit. Mrs Smith had popped a note through the door stating she could help, but he had never asked.

Try to picture yourself as a professional who is on duty and receives the call from Mrs Smith. You look up your records and identify that there has been no previous involvement by your 'department', and no known needs or risk assessment, or recorded diagnosis or case formulation. Before you decide that you need to obtain more information try to answer these two questions.

1. Peter does not have a diagnosis, although you suspect an autistic spectrum disorder. From the information you have, what would make you consider this diagnosis? You will need to be able to highlight these if looking for further information or support for Peter.
2. What other underlying explanations or causes (including another mental disorder) could this behaviour be due to?

Further information is then obtained from a colleague who has a note of a contact with his mother from some years back, which is on her file:

> Peter has always lived at home with his mother. Peter has a daily routine, which includes getting up when his mother brings him a cup of tea. He gets dressed, and his mother opens the post while she waits for him to get ready to help with the chores around the house. Peter always does the vacuuming, while his mother washes the clothes and does the ironing. Peter would then help his mother with the food shopping, carrying the bags and putting the shopping away. Peter enjoys his mother's cooking; she always has a special dish for each day. Friday is fish and chip night. His mother would give Peter the money and he would get the fish and chips for himself and his mother.

3. *Again, what else have you seen here to suggest an autistic problem and/or another way of explaining what is happening here.*

Later we will come back to this account and consider what additional information the reader might seek and also what short-term, 'immediate', action might need to be taken.

Discussion of possible responses and what each means or could mean.

Q1. Peter's story is quite typical of the pattern of an older adult who continues to live with a surviving parent in the original family home until ill health or even death forces social care agencies or other authorities (or volunteers) to step in. Peter has fixed habits and rituals, and is unable to change these when circumstance requires it. In the past, one suspects that such accounts led to long-term hospitalization within mental health services. Recent experience where autism is a confirmed diagnosis is that such individuals with a period of social care input can be supported to bridge the gap by adapting and learning to use independent living skills that heretofore they left to a parent or carer to provide. When asked why they don't wash, tidy, pay bills, shop for food they will typically say 'there is no need to—she does everything'.

Q2. Of course, this could also be a case of a man with mild intellectual disability who is able to communicate verbally, but is very dependent for basic care needs. Needless to say, depression and psychosis or, rarely, in the older dependent adult, early onset cognitive impairment need to be considered as alternative explanations. Hence, the importance of an assessment process led by a professional with expertise in all of these areas of behavioural difficulty in adulthood. Physical health should also be part of any assessment.

Case Study F

A referral to an adult mental health team from a GP:

> Dear Team
>
> I would be grateful for your urgent assessment of this 25-year-old young man. His mother has reported him to me as he is depressed and talking of self-harm. His computer has just been impounded by the police on suspicion of downloading child pornography and he is on police bail.
>
> His mother describes him as being a late talker who has always been a loner, who never fitted in at school. He did well at primary school. He always liked routine and order and was bullied in his secondary school. He went to a single sex boarding school at the age of 10 due to his parents travel abroad. There was apparently trouble at school due to him getting drunk and he was threatened with suspension, but this did not happen again. He has not had any contact with friends from boarding school since leaving.
>
> He left with good examination grades. He went to university to do Geology, but dropped out due to unhappiness. He could not cope with the halls of residence and was not capable of living independently in self-catering halls. He is currently looking to go to university while living at home.
>
> I have found him an odd young man who looks very flat and depressed. He says he is not sleeping—being unable to get to sleep due to worry. He is eating though. He says he does not look forward to the future. He does not answer questions about the police allegations, but seems unconcerned about them. He talks of suicide in a very matter of fact manner. I am seriously concerned.

Q1. The young man does not have a diagnosis, but from the information you have what would make you consider an autistic spectrum disorder?

Q2. What other kinds of explanations could there be for this behaviour?

Discussion of possible responses and what each means or could mean.

Q1. Possible pointers to a late recognition of autism include being isolated at school and 'not fitting in', then dropping out early from a degree course, not managing independent living in spite of signs of good educational achievement. Liking routine and order, and being bullied in school are also alerting signals. Getting into trouble with the law with use of a computer, including cybercrime, is being suggested as having a link with autism, but not yet been researched. The account suggests longer-term problems with no period of deterioration or of 'onset', which points more towards a neurodevelopmental and, thus, lifelong difficulty.

Q2. An alternative explanation that must be considered is either a developing depressive disorder or a psychotic condition. People with autism can sometimes forget to eat and can neglect the need for sleep and be found to spend much of the day asleep in their rooms, therefore missing college lessons, work start times, etc. Comorbidity between depression and autism, which is very much an issue for late childhood and adult life, can make assessment complex and difficult, a topic to be returned to later.

Case Study G

A referral to an adult mental health team from a GP:

> Dear Team
>
> I would be grateful for your urgent assessment of this 20-year-old young man. His father has reported him to me because he was not leaving his room to eat and I visited to find his room barricaded.
>
> His parents are from India, and have lived in this country since before his birth. He has not been seen by us before. He is described by his father as a studious boy who initially did well at university, but had some problems and has returned home. Here, he has related most to his mother, but she is currently in India due to her own mother being ill.
>
> We have no record of previous contact with services. He was apparently always a loner who worked hard in his room and only came downstairs to eat. He did not join in family gatherings, except under extreme pressure from his parents. His father thinks he has friends, but talks to them on the Internet.
>
> When he went to university to study mathematics he apparently did well, but got into trouble as he exposed himself to some female students in his block. He was asked to leave and has been at home for the last 9 months.
>
> He has been isolating himself in his room increasingly since return from university. His father tells me that his wife always cooked him food different to the rest of the family and, more recently, he has only eaten pre-prepared food using the microwave in his room. He has been doing his own washing, but insists that he takes it wet up to his room and dries it there.
>
> His father says that since being back from university his son would walk around the house with a mask on his face if he did not tell him to take it off. He will go out, but has not done so for several weeks. His father has not seen him outside his room for over a week, although he hears him regularly jumping and shouting in his room at various times of the day and night. He does have a bathroom attached to his bedroom.
>
> I have tried to visit, but found the stairs to his room piled with his items from university, all sealed in plastic. He refused to open the door to see me and told me to go away when I tried to speak through the door.

Q1. The young man does not have a diagnosis, but from the information you have what would make you consider an autistic spectrum disorder?

Q2. What other kinds of explanations could there be for this behaviour?

Discussion of possible responses and what each means or could mean.

Q1. Behaviour with members of the opposite sex (or with others to whom an individual is sexually attracted) that gives rise to concern is not unusual in both younger men and women on the autism spectrum. (As well as giving offence to others, as important is their vulnerability to exploitation by others—this applies particularly to young women on the autism spectrum who are also poor at recognizing signals and at knowing how to get out of situations they do not want to be in.) In this account we also see behaviour that draws the attention of others in the household to this individual, suggesting that he is unaware of the impact of his behaviour on others. Cultural factors might explain why there is no record of previous contact with services.[5]

Q2. The account at first suggests an acute issue that may require urgent action, possibly with the onset of a psychotic illness. This would not be an unusual reason for a family doctor to turn to specialist mental health services in relation to such a young man. The mention by the family doctor that the young man's bedroom was barricaded may be a misunderstanding—at least the alternative explanation of cluttering so that only the occupant is able to enter and leave, should be considered. Collecting objects with no intrinsic purpose leading to clutter is a common problem in autism. With the onset of adult life, a parent (usually the mother) may find it is no longer possible to clear out clutter without encountering very strong resistance and even violence from her affected offspring. Siblings, where one is behaviourally disabled, can also engage in quite odd behaviours in order to cope with having to live together (we have not been told if there are siblings in this household). The account also points to a strong possibility that an autism presentation is being exacerbated by the development of depression. It will be all the more important in such cases to check early development before assuming that autism is the underlying problem, which it might not be. Physical health should also be looked into as local services may not know about him.

Concluding thoughts and reflections on developing awareness of autism in adulthood

There may be readers for whom the realization is developing that autism is a condition that they may sometimes have missed, perhaps because the symptoms and behaviours were masked in some way and because thoughts turned to other diagnostic labels. An example might be the term '*misaphonia*',

---

[5] The author's practice is in the city of Leicester, where white European people are a minority of the population, but make up most of the referrals from the city to this adult 'Asperger' diagnostic clinic.

which is a distressingly heightened sensitivity to specific sounds that is also one of the commoner symptoms of sensory sensitivity in autism, which will be covered in detail in Chapters 3, 7, and 8. A second example is hoarding, which is a not unusual component of the rigidity also seen in some cases of autism, covered in the same chapters. Ideally, we would have learnt these things as medical students and as doctors in further training.

The reader might ask themselves were these learning exercises all that difficult? How did you get on with identifying possible features of autism in these accounts? Has this complemented your alertness to possible signals of other kinds of mental health issues, and the possibility of either co-existing developmental problems or, indeed, long-term developmental problems that only come to wider attention, which may explain an initial presenting problem?

A basic knowledge base, as we work forward, is the early psychological and particularly social development of the person in such cases. It was noted, in the last case study, that this person's later emerging difficulties could be due to a gradual onset of mental illness or to long-standing autism, or to some combination of both. In adult psychiatry we are not used to dwelling in much detail on early development, in the sense that our colleagues in paediatrics do. Faced with such cases, the hallmark of a correct diagnosis is the early developmental history (Chapter 7). For many, well established in the practice of psychiatry in adulthood, learning the skills and the knowledge required to conduct a developmental history is going to be a particular challenge. Observations of early development, are said to vary from the *typical* ('typical'[6] is a word that some child specialists prefer to the word 'normal'), to the *atypical* (which for some is also the preferred term for alterations from normal development). Underlying psychological theories will be touched upon, although these are still very much in development, but sufficiently so to exploit their value in understanding the nature of autism, if only from the point of view of possible metaphors that could be helpful in practice.

---

[6] The term 'neurotypical', pleural 'neurotypicals' occurs frequently both in the developmental literature and also in the writings of people on the autism spectrum. These are not universally accepted terms.

Chapter 3

Development of behaviour and functioning (with hindsight)

Background

> 'Autism is a developmental condition affecting the way the brain processes information. It occurs in varying levels of severity and is a lifelong condition; autistic children become autistic adults.'[1]

Definitions of autism, the history of the development of the concept, the experience of it from the perspective of adults with the diagnosis, all provide the underpinning 'data' we need in adult psychiatry to be equipped to understand and explore autism. Before describing how development follows a different course in autism, we require some consideration of what processes might underpin the condition and how to investigate them. Unfortunately, far less underpinning knowledge is available to us and, therefore, less is known and understood about autism.

The role of the phenomenological approach to understanding autism

The late and widely lauded neurologist, Oliver Sacks, argued that 'to understand the autistic individual, nothing less than a total biography will do' (Chapter 4). The busy clinician need not be daunted by this idealistic proposition. In practice, a few minutes spent asking an older mother about the early childhood development of her, now young, adult, offspring can be illuminating and highly informative, sometimes bringing a clear demonstration of an obvious case of autism. The diagnostic criteria for autism (Chapter 1) are thus part developmental, but when applied to the adult, they are also part phenomenological.

---

[1] Reproduced with permission from The National Autistic Society

Until now, assessment methods have been based on those appropriate to and feasible in childhood. Guided (expert) observation captures and codes behaviour in different (varied) real life settings that an autistic child may find challenging, such as play and peer interaction. Interviews are also carried out separately with parents and teachers and other carers, with regard to longer-term perspectives on the development of the child. These methods continue to be applied in early adult life. Clinicians developing diagnostic services for the older adult and the elderly are discovering that reliable early life developmental data can be difficult or impossible to obtain. Direct observation (Chapter 9) of behaviour is limited to what is practical, usually a 1:1 interview, lasting more or less than 1 hour. (For many with the condition any longer could be intolerable to endure, particularly if there is intellectual disability).

Autism specialists have yet to explore and publish findings on the use of the methods that adult mental health professionals rely on. As the reader knows, these methods are based on the exploration of the personal experience of the person with autism, that is, these are substantially based on the phenomenological approach (Chapter 8). In Chapter 4 we will see examples of personal descriptions of the experiences and of the world perspectives of persons with autism, which could also inform us about its recognition and its assessment (discussed in subsequent chapters).

The phenomenological approach, and other approaches used in adult mental health assessment, also rely on concepts of the underlying disorder, however unclear or, indeed, speculative. In the case of psychosis, it is necessary to have an understanding of the sensory modalities in order to be able to discuss with a potential patient abnormal experiences, such as hallucination or lesser perceptual variations such as depersonalization, as a physician would discuss any medical condition, and without any stigmatizing implications. An understanding of memory, intelligence, and cognitive processing, are important in exploring abnormal inference, such as delusion. Similar principles apply to the understanding of emotion and of abnormal mood. Some of these are experiences that we can all identify in ourselves, making it relatively straightforward to discuss them empathically with our patients.

Theories of abnormal (or atypical) psychological development

Behaviours and experiences observed in autism, in part, may be explained by putative underlying developmental deficits. We have already begun to explore these in the previous chapter, where we considered possible characteristics and traits that might alert us to the possibility of autism in someone we know or in a request for advice from a colleague. It is essential to keep in mind at all times that most of these are just theories—some of which are partly supported and some of which are refuted by experimental evidence, which we need not go into in detail about here, there being excellent sources elsewhere for the interested reader (Amaral et al. 2011; Tantam, 2012). (See also the section on recommended general and further reading at the end of Chapter 15.)

Knowledge and research design

Before looking at what underpinning research may be able to tell us about autism, a moment on study design may be helpful. Studying autism scientifically is particularly challenging. At present, of course, it is not possible to study the brain directly *in vivo*. Biological material outside the brain may give some indication of underlying mechanisms, but we cannot be sure of its biological relevance. Neurophysiology and neuroimaging are also indirect, although there is much optimism about the potential of the latter, in particular. (Animal model research may provide alternative ways of testing hypotheses but findings may not be applicable to patients).

A substantial proportion of autism research studies compare persons (mainly children), meeting criteria for autism, with others who are 'normal'. These research findings need careful interpretation. If the 'others', i.e. the controls, are 'normal', how can we be sure that any difference between the groups is due to autism specifically? Better comparisons, seen less often, use additional controls that include individuals with other abnormalities of brain functioning, such as ADHD, uncomplicated intellectual disability. Relatively few studies compare more with less severe forms of autism, on the basis that any associated factor will be related to severity or complexity of autism.

Major differences between research experimental groups also raise the issue of researcher bias. As the autism phenotype needs to be assessed in both groups, if it is all too obvious to a trained researcher what behaviours individuals with autism exhibit, it may be very difficult to carry out truly blinded testing. Good research papers will discuss these limitations and how they have been addressed, wherever possible.

Theories of underlying cognitive difficulties

In order to understand the presenting features in autism, it is helpful to first consider what are currently thought to be the underlying cognitive difficulties, namely, impaired theory of mind, lack of central coherence and

> **Box 3.1 Psychological concepts thought to give rise to the behaviours that underlie autism include difficulties with the following areas of cognitive functioning**
>
> - Theory of mind.
> - The ability to see the world as others do.
> - Central coherence.
> - The ability to see beyond the detail, to the bigger picture within.
> - Executive functioning.
> - The ability to sequence, organize, and plan.

difficulties in executive functioning, each of which need to be considered briefly, and which are thought to be the main difficulties that underlie autism (Box 3.1).

Theory of mind ability

Theory of mind (TOM) refers to the ability to attribute mental states (including beliefs, intents, desires, knowledge, and pretence) to oneself and other people, and to understand that others have beliefs, desires, and intentions that are different from one's own. It is an ability that develops gradually over time—not a light switch that comes on suddenly at a particular age.

The best known test used by psychologists to demonstrate difficulties in this area is the 'Sally Ann Test' (Baron-Cohen, 1985). The examiner enacts a scene with two dolls. The child being tested watches the two dolls in a room; their names are Sally and Anne. Sally has a basket and Anne has a box. Sally has a marble that she places in her basket; Sally then leaves the room. Anne who has nothing in her box takes Sally's marble and places it in her box. Sally returns to the room. The child watching this is asked by the experimenter "where will Sally look for the marble"? If the child is developing normally ('typically') it will say, "Sally will look where it was when she left the room", a reasonable belief that shows development of theory of mind. An autistic child will say where the marble is now—a true, but an unreasonable belief.

However, a note of caution may be included here, as older and more able individuals with autism can use their intellect to work out how to 'pass the test' when challenged. Difficulties in this area probably are better demonstrated by enquiring how a person functions in real-life social situations,

What is this?

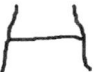

Fig. 3.1 A test of central coherence (1).

where they are required to apply their understanding in an uncontrolled and unrehearsed setting, noting the degree of extra effort this costs the person. A tendency towards 'mind blindness'[2] will often persist into adult life, and give rise to social difficulties and isolation or social exclusion because the affected person either cannot or is simply not motivated to make the effort to see how other people relate to one another.

Central coherence abilities

Central coherence is the ability to assimilate all the information at hand, along with using relevant prior knowledge, to see the 'bigger picture,' or *gestalt*. It is a necessary process to allow information to be taken in context. Difficulties in this domain mean that people with autism naturally tend to focus more on minor details/think about things in the smallest possible parts, but 'cannot see the wood for the trees' (Happe, 2006). Consequently, they may miss important information or misinterpret situations due to failing to understand the full circumstance.

Let us use an example to illustrate central coherence. In the first of the following three diagrams what do you think the symbol in Fig. 3.1 represents? Then look at Figs. 3.2 and 3.3. The additional information provides the context needed to answer the question; in autism context tends to be ignored.

Note, however, that ease with focusing on detail may be advantageous in the more technically demanding activities needed by scientists and engineers. In many social situations it can be very disadvantageous.

Executive functioning abilities

Executive functioning is employed for activities such as sequencing, organizing, and planning ahead. Lack of awareness and internal monitoring of time and space in people with autism can render them less likely to think in a sequential framework, and thus understand and predict the world. As a

---
[2] A term for general TOM difficulties, possibly introduced by Simon Baron-Cohen.

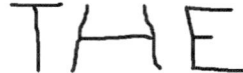

Fig. 3.2 A test of central coherence (2).

consequence, even those who are highly intellectually able, can struggle to attend to 'day-to-day' functions, such as scheduling routine responsibilities, keeping up with household chores, and managing their money, as well as more major challenges, such as coping with the unexpected.

However, impaired executive functioning is also observed in other conditions seen by psychiatrists, notably schizophrenia (and psychosis more generally) and in ADHD.

Underpinning science

Psychological functions thought to underlie autism, which have come from the field of cognitive and neuropsychology, parallel a welter of more neurobiological-based research. For comprehensive reviews Digby Tantam's impressive monograph is recommend, written by an adult clinician and psychotherapist, with an integrated span of a complex literature, thoroughly and comprehensively reviewed and synthesized (Tantam, 2012). Also recommended, as an entry point to a range of different approaches by different research groups, is Amaral and his colleagues overview of the science of autism, albeit, almost exclusively based on childhood studies (Amaral et al. 2011).

Underpinning neurobiological research

A recent comprehensive review of autism discusses the possible underlying neurobiology of autism (Lai et al. 2014). More sceptical arguments should also be considered (Waterhouse et al. 2016).

There is growing research interest in the idea that brain abnormalities underlying autism may be partly explained by abnormalities in neural connectivity, rather than by abnormalities located to specific brain areas. Indeed, very many different brain areas have been implicated in autism

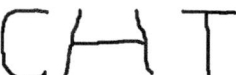

Fig. 3.3 A test of central coherence (3).

(Tantam, 2012). Early brain overgrowth from 6 to 18 months of age has also been widely studied. Alterations in both serotonin and γ-aminobutyric-acid (GABA) systems have been reported quite consistently.

There are various neurological theories of autism, but one that seems particularly compelling and which may have some heuristic value in clinical practice is mirror neurone theory.

Mirror neurones—a compellingly attractive theory

Although controversial, and not universally accepted, the concept of mirror neurones represents a paradigm for difficulties in theory of mind ability, which clinicians find attractive in developing some sense or understanding of what may, in part, be the neural basis for autism.

Imitation is a fundamental mechanism underlying early learning— specifically spontaneous imitation, as seen in the first 2 years of an infant's life, thought to play a critical role in learning language and social values. There is some evidence that deficits in these abilities are associated with autism, although not all neuroscientists accept this or its value as a worthwhile line of research. Mirroring is also found in other primates and, indeed, in other species (making it open to invasive investigation that would be unethical in human subjects). The chapter by Marco Icabone in Amaral's textbook (Iacoboni, 2011) provides an accessible overview, although the serious student should include more up-to-date papers.

Developmental differences characteristic of the autism phenotype

Autism is fundamentally a disorder of psychological development and particularly in the social and communicational aspects. In order to learn how to obtain a developmental history (Chapter 7) we need to spend some time describing the threshold between the typical and the atypical, that is, between the normal and the abnormal in development. The remainder of this chapter is devoted to describing these developmental differences in some detail (Box 3.2).

The remainder of this chapter is also inspired by the work of Dr Lorna Wing, and by the continuation of that work by Dr Judith Gould, Dr Susan Leekam, and others who worked most closely with her. Lorna led the way in drawing attention to how essential this knowledge base is to a clear understanding of autism. The following descriptions are based on essential components of development that can often be assessed many years later in adulthood, with the help of a suitable informant.

Box 3.2 Underlying developmental differences specific to autism

Infancy and the first 12 months of life
- Attention and interests
- Joint referencing
- Early signs of social awareness

Language and communication
- Speech development
- Reciprocity in communication

Body language (non-verbal communication)
- Facial expression
- Use of gesture

Social interaction
- Social awareness
- Preferences for others
- Friendship

Eye contact
Quality, use of gaze.

Imagination and pretence
- Make believe play.
- Repertoire of interests.

Bodily movements
Stereotypy and mannerisms such as tip toe walking.

Sensory differences
Responses to under- and over-stimulation.

Proximal sensory stimulation

- Handling of objects.
- Self-stimulation.

Response to sounds

Attraction to or distressful reaction.

Response to visual stimuli and other sensory differences

- Fascination with different sensory experiences.
- Distress triggered by normal stimuli.

Routines and resistance to change

- Collecting.
- Maintenance of routines and sameness in surroundings.
- Resistance to change.

Behaviour problems in childhood and adulthood

- Behaviour at home and in public places.
- In childhood and now in adulthood.

In Chapter 7 we learn about obtaining a developmental history from an informant, who has closely known and observed our adult patient since birth and infancy. This is based on the assessment tool, the Diagnostic Interview for Social and communication Disorders (DISCO; Wing, 1993, 2000; Leekam et al. 2002; Wing et al. 2002). The reader will explore and learn how to ask about differences in early development, how to interpret what informants (or child records) tell us, which questions are easy and which are harder for parents and observers to reply to.

Developmental differences, particularly those that seem to more clearly characterize the autism phenotype, are listed in Box 3.2. They follow the structure adopted by Wing and Gould in the DISCO. The present chapter will conclude with a reminder of indicators of general development (motor coordination, self-care, independence, etc.), which are also important in the assessment of need in autism.

Here, we describe some of the underlying developmental differences in autism, noting that it is not a comprehensive list.

Infancy and the first 12 months of life

Infants begin to communicate from the moment of child birth (some mothers would argue that communication begins in the womb). Needs are communicated through the voice and facial expression and suckling. A great deal emerges in the first months and in the first year of life. Parents (and grandparents) are delighted when the infant begins to engage through gaze, looking at the carer.

Difficulties in eye gaze are a key characteristic of autism throughout the entire life cycle and can be observed by the clinician encountering the adult patient. We will expand on this later, when we come to look at the DISCO in Chapter 7, and consider eye gaze differences, suggestive of autism, compared with those described in conditions like anxiety, depression, and severe mental illness (Chapter 9).

Gesture also begins to play a part. The child indicates that it wants to be picked up by a carer by gazing at her (or him) and holding out its arms (or responds to the carer showing similar signs of picking up the infant).

A particularly complex, but thought to be crucial development, which is often extremely difficult for parents to recall many years later, is the concept of joint referencing or sharing of interest. Here, the child will point to objects or events of interest, and then look to the mother or carer in order to share the interest. Sharing may even be literal—as in picking up an object and offering it to the care giver (such as offering food on a spoon, once the child has the necessary motor skills to do so).

Language and communication

Until recently, under DSM-IV and ICD-10, significant delay in language development was marked out as the dividing line between 'childhood autism', on the one hand, and 'Asperger syndrome and high functioning autism' on the other (ICD-10; World Health Organization, 1993). Some of these are covered below (Box 3.3), under development of communication and understanding. In the context of autism, a number of specific features of language development difference or delay are thought to be 'pathognomonic'.

When assessing adults, mainly with relatively normal (typical) development of communication ability, it is only occasionally that one observes or hears relatives describing echoing (frequent repetition of words, phrases), mixing up of pronouns, using words with special (idiosyncratic) meanings. However, for colleagues who are responsible for consulting with adults with

Box 3.3 Differences in development of language and communication pointing to autism

- Delayed echoing (repetitive use of words or phrases).
- Mixing up pronouns.
- Repetitive speech (same topics constantly repeated).
- Unusual or peculiar use of words (special meanings).
- Literal understanding.
- Appreciation of humour.
- Ability to hold a two-way conversation.
- Tone of voice.

intellectual disability (i.e. 'learning disabilities'), these unusual uses of language are seen frequently. Indeed, much of the use of language in intellectually disabled adults exhibits these characteristics. In the more able adult population, literal understanding and a lack of appreciation of the humour of others often stand out and, indeed, mark some of their most important day-to-day difficulties, which undermine social functioning and integration.

Literal understanding

Literal understanding difficulties and a lack of appreciation of humour are often referred to as difficulties in the pragmatic aspects of language and understanding. When the meaning of certain words depends on the circumstances (or context) in which they are expressed, understanding what is actually being referred to is more likely to raise difficulties for someone with autism or, indeed, for someone with autistic traits, as in the broader autism phenotype. This is also a good example of why autism or autistic traits can be viewed as differences, rather than as deficits in ability.[3]

Difficulties involving over-literal understanding can be assessed both via a caregiver (parent; Chapter 7) and through direct observation (Chapter 9).

---

[3] More research is needed in this area because we do not yet know whether such differences are part of a non-specific population continuum or represent a characteristic of greater clinical significance; the clinician will therefore want to know how much this impacts negatively (or positively) on the patient's life and circumstances, for good or ill.

The distinction between explicit and implicit use of language may be helpful here. An example may be used to illustrate this. Engineers, scientists, and thankfully aircraft passenger pilots and air traffic controllers, abhor any ambiguity of meaning in the words others chose to use. People with quite different (i.e. 'typical') inclinations soon find such explicit, direct, or literal communication tiresome and rigid. In contrast, in the world of diplomacy, great value is placed on the ability to choose words that are not direct, the meaning of which is implied and depends on particular circumstances. What the listener chooses to hear or to 'take' may encourage the fostering of further discussion or conversation until, eventually, at such time as the participants feel able to confront more difficult issues, greater directness may be tolerable and necessary.

Adults on the autism spectrum find such lack of explicitness in communication far more difficult. Digressing further, this may be why there appear to be more such persons settling down, living, and working in geographic areas in which 'high-tech' science and engineering literally dominate the local landscape. It should not surprise the reader to find that assessing these characteristics can be difficult, perhaps more so, if an informant also finds indirect, implicit use of language problematic (Chapter 7).[4]

Two-way interaction

Problems with two-way interaction are another crucial aspect of communication that is all too common an issue for the otherwise able adult, who may be autistic. Flexible, two-way, reciprocal interaction, the ability to give and take, respond to what the other says (rather than to rigidly dominate the subject of discussion, refusing to go along with whatever direction the flow of communication takes), are often referred to with terms such as 'conversation' and chat, or 'chit-chat'. Observant autistic adults, openly willing to cast a critical eye on their neurotypical (non-autistic) peers, refer to this as 'talking about nothing' and as 'pointless chatter'. This is one of the reasons they greatly dislike social occasions; they find it difficult to do this and prefer to be 'doing something useful', 'talking about' something tangible, and thus, although wanting some social contact, often choose seemingly self-imposed isolation. The typical two-way interaction that runs deeper than this—utterance, followed by response, followed by another utterance that reflects what has been said, or communicated—rarely comes easily to the autistic person, who will often lapse into silence unless asked a question

---

[4] Different versions of the same language, e.g. American and English usage of English words, may also cause similar difficulties.

directly. We can even observe two-way interaction parallels in other mammalian species in their, almost exclusively, non-verbal modes of communication, including sniffing, looking, turning away, back scratching—i.e. give and take, give and take, all seemingly pointless, but all contributing towards social integration and cohesion. Assessing this aspect of communication can also be challenging, as we shall see later.

Vocal intonation

Vocal intonation refers to modulation of voice, volume, variation in pitch and vocal emphasis (in autism some speak so quietly it is hard to hear what is being said, others so loudly that embarrassment may result from unwitting disclosure to strangers of personal information). It may be easier to remember to think of and take note of this as another gap in the person's ability to see and understand things from the point of view of others, i.e. taking others into account. In some cases, it may stand out as a rather metallic sounding monotony of intonation; in others odd and unexpected increases in vocal pitch—the speaker seemingly unaware of its impact on others.

Non-verbal communication

Body language (non-verbal communication) comprises of the use of gesture and variation in facial expression. (It may be helpful to think of these as sitting alongside the previous topic, vocal intonation, which is also symbolic, rather than direct or literal, although gesture can be symbolic and informative). Variations in body language can be observed directly by the clinician also (Chapter 9). It is also important to collect the observations of others, based on substantial periods of time going back into childhood (Chapter 7), because a short period of direct observation (in one's consulting room) may not represent the person's ongoing style of communication. It may also be that the use of gesture varies according to the level of emotional arousal; in autism emotional arousal tends to switch rather suddenly from low to high, whereas in the typically developed adult change in arousal levels is much more gradual. Informants may therefore describe observing a general lack of gesture punctuated by periods of extreme or exaggerated use of gesture.[5] The typical consulting room may represent the former mode of functioning only, which may mislead the unaware clinician.

---

[5] There are also different types of gesture that can be thought of in terms of a hierarchy—emotional, emphatic, conventional, instrumental, informational, and descriptive gesture. It is not just whether or not someone uses gestures, but how and at what level of complexity.

Non-verbal communication also occupies the dividing line between literal, direct, communication, and pragmatics—knowing the intended meaning, rather than what appears to be communicated at surface level. It helps us to pick up how the person feels today, which helps us to choose and judge whether today is a good time or not to ask for a favour: 'it's not *what* you say, but *how* you say it that matters'.

The extent to which people make use of body language, and rely on it to understand what others mean, varies enormously between persons, and between contexts and cultures. Some regard deficits in non-verbal communication as the core sign of the condition. One of the problems with that view is that it seems to be at variance with a gradually dawning realization that some able adults may be able to *learn* how to appear to use non-verbal communication, perhaps more so in able women than men (Brugha et al. 2016). 'Faking it' is not easy. Nor, seemingly, is it easy for persons who are normally adept at communicating, non-verbally, to switch it off (literally by sitting on their hands).

Social interaction

Deficits in social interaction abilities are especially important to any consideration of a diagnosis on the autism spectrum. If absent (following adequate assessment), autism can be confidently ruled out. If present, a wide range of other behavioural conditions, some of them common comorbidities of autism, may be possible explanations (see Chapter 10). Before discussing another key topic, friendship development and maintenance, key aspects of social interaction need to be considered first.

Ability to react to the feelings of others

Emotional empathy is the ability to recognize others feelings, and to know instinctively how to react and respond to others. A lack of this ability is a quite common symptom. It may appear to occur in adults who have been exposed to much emotional abuse and/or neglect in earlier life; therefore, they may be observed now by others as only reacting to others feelings and emotions, when they are strongly and obviously expressed, suggesting a secondary effect on behaviour. It is important to ask the person themselves about this and not just to rely on the observations of others. Patients may describe being able to understand how others feel, but just not being able to react. The term 'being tight lipped', thought to be part of English male culture, comes to mind. Parents sometimes find it hard to remember when their child developed sensitivity to the feelings of others, and this ability can continue to emerge and improve well into adulthood (i.e. possibly beyond the age of 25 years).

Lack of interest in age peers

Lack of interest in age peers is especially telling. The parent may describe how their child preferred to spend time and play on its own, rather than in the company of others its own age. Their child may even have become very distressed when introduced for the first time to the company of others their own age. A characteristic sign is observed in the child or adult who finds the company of people significantly older or younger than they are easier. The young child may find it preferable to spend time with teachers (going to the teacher's room or the library) during school break times. The older individual may find the company of children not just tolerable, but much easier. Surprisingly, many older teenage women on the autism spectrum, one has observed, chose to train in infant and child care (and sometimes are very good at learning and following the required procedures).[6] Unfortunately, an adult who shows a preference for the company of children may be misunderstood.

Passivity

The autistic child and younger adult may also display a striking passivity in their interaction with their peers. (S)he may be overly vulnerable to their influence, such that he or she engages, seemingly willingly, in behaviour that they would never take part in of their own volition. Being socially naive, they will often be the ones to get caught, when the more alert, neurotypical members of the peer group run away, so that the misdemeanour is attributed to the autistic child by an authority figure. Occasionally, such behaviours by an autistic individual have led to charges of criminal behaviour. Although this feature of development is rare it is very striking when observed. Most parents asked this question of their child will describe quite the opposite observation— their child is so stubborn and rigid that no one can get them to do their bidding.

Lorna's Wing's team referred to such social *passivity* as one of three sub-types of social impairment, the other two being, '*aloof*', and '*active-but-odd*' (Wing and Gould 1979).

Other social functioning differences

Other social deficits include a tendency to make one-sided approaches to others, approaching others on their own terms without taking account of the other's feelings or needs, adopting a seemingly superior attitude to others, even being strikingly polite and formal with people they know well.

---

[6] Thus, the child carer escapes the scrutiny of adults and is free to behave unselfconsciously.

Lack of social understanding for developmental age is quite a common problem that can be particularly stressful for parents when out in public with their child who, for example, may make tactless comments and behave in a naive inappropriate way in the company of other adults.[7] This is one of the few aspects of social development that seems to improve with adulthood (although this may require a conscious effort on the part of the individual, which may bring a cost in terms of reduced time spent in public settings).

Friendship

Problems with making friends are very common, almost ubiquitous in autism, although autism is not the only reason for this problem (see later chapters). When we discuss the assessment of early development the point will be made that autistic adults, when asked if they have friends, often will say 'yes'. As the reader will see, the examiner should not take this at face value. It may also be possible to assess this area of difficulty through direct interview, but it does require careful attention to the best way to put such questions.

What seems to underlie difficulties in friendship formation, which should be consistently observable throughout the life course from the earliest days? One of the frequent deficits is in reciprocity—in give and take (see previously). The autistic individual lacks an interest in and a *curiosity* about the concerns of the life of their friend/s and, particularly, the *feelings* of others. Anniversaries are forgotten (unless reminders are programmed into an organizer, which may lead to over-formal observation of the obligation to note the event). Favours and gifts received are not reciprocated. Interaction tends to be confined to a few shared interests. Face-to-face contact is notably infrequent without a reasonable explanation. Chit chat is not part of their interaction. A good-looking autistic teenager may also be popular for a while because of skills in playing a new computer game. They may attract a peer group following, who are prepared to overlook their general lack of natural affiliative behaviours, albeit temporarily. When separation comes, with moves to work or further education, the autistic individual fails to make the effort to keep in touch, although some of their peers do so with ease and thus develop firmer longer-term friendships.

Experiences of bullying

It is very common for boys to describe bullying experiences, particularly in the teen years but, sometimes, much earlier. If autistic, the child may not have known how to challenge or control this. Often parents will also know

---

[7] Blurting out inappropriate verbal interjections may also be an alerting sign to possible ADHD.

about it and, sometimes, will have complained to the child's school (where most instances occur). Bullying is far too common to be a salient predictor of autism (but the nature and quality of bullying and the child's response to it may reveal more). Bullying may also continue into the workplace in adulthood (this is more unusual and probably a more useful indicator of possible autistic difficulties). Neighbourhood bullying may lead to the person having to move accommodation.[8] Safeguarding issues may arise (Chapter 13).

These remarks reflect the historical nature of any assessment of early childhood development—we are looking back into the past—these observations may not be applicable now and in the future as society evolves and previous gender stereotypes alter.

Eye contact, gaze

Problems with gaze and eye contact are believed by many autism experts to be essential to the diagnosis. There may be gender differences in the expression of these characteristics; women may be more capable than men in engaging, seemingly normally, in this way. Poor eye contact is also a feature of some forms of mental illness in adults, but in such cases eye contact will have been normal before the condition developed. Abnormal eye contact may also occur for purely physical or medical reasons, such as untreated amblyopia. At its simplest level, autistic persons have poor eye contact and many will also describe it as being very difficult to look at another person's eyes. One indication of poor use of eye gaze is a tendency to stare—to look too long into the other person's eyes, which can be very intimidating (and for the medical observer, the first trigger to thinking—'I wonder might this person be on the autism spectrum?')

If poor eye gaze is picked up in childhood, the child may have been successfully trained to look at the nose, forehead, or some other facial feature. They may also have been taught, if unsure who or what to look at, to look down (a signal of submission, which is non-threatening). Such ostensibly successful training early in life may mean that a continuing autism in adulthood is overlooked or is regarded as not being severe, the affected person, meanwhile, struggling to keep to those early life instructions, at some personal cost in ongoing effort. More will be said about what to watch out for in the chapters on developmental assessment (Chapters 7 and 9 in particular). Sometimes spotting these areas of difficulty depends on accruing a good deal of clinical experience.

---

[8] This is something that housing officials and professional tenancy organization staff can be taught to be aware of, in order to support those adults who are vulnerable in this way (Chapter 14).

Imagination and pretence

The normal child will begin to engage in make believe play, possibly from as early as 18 months of age. They may conceal it from adults as they grow older (Dunn 2004). There seems to be a natural in-built tendency to make up activities that often correspond to a form of adult behaviour, such as dressing up and feeding babies or little children, putting them to sleep, etc. At a slightly older age it may be pretending to be soldiers, police and robbers, etc. Innocent looking objects, such as a rough piece of wood, may suddenly depict instead a weapon—a sword or a gun. Dressing up does not require obtaining precise replicas or copies of the garb of the role to be engaged in. The distinction between imagination and imitation, as we shall see in the chapter on developmental assessment, is important. In a group of children, one or two may 'write the script', others may go along with this and be content to 'follow directions' (it is the latter amongst whom possible cases of autism or autistic traits may be observed).

Lorna's Wing's criteria for autism include deficits in imagination. That clearly requires an assessment of child development, often impossible in the older adult who has, until then, gone unrecognized, because there is no one else able to recall and describe it. In the adult the ability to see things as others do, and to be inventive, particularly in social contexts, will be the equivalent ground on which to base ongoing assessment. The ability to anticipate the consequences of one's actions and the ability to foresee how others may behave in response to one's actions or to what one might say also requires imaginative ability. Failure to anticipate consequences can give rise to significant difficulties for an adult with unrecognized autism. It can also be a factor to be considered in advising a Court in relation to a criminal charge.

Adults on the autism spectrum often feel a strong need to plan meticulously for anything novel or different in the future, such as to go to a place that is unfamiliar, or to engage in activity or contact with others who they have never met before. (Free online mapping has made planning much easier, as has the entire repository of information on the Internet). Most of the rest of the neurotypical population will be quite relaxed about most future events, being content to 'take things in their stride', except, of course, for a crucially important future event, such as a key job interview, or a crucial learning or work presentation.

Lack of imagination in childhood can also manifest itself in a narrow repertoire of interests. The child (and this may continue in adulthood) is only interested in reading about or viewing material on specific kinds of facts, with little interest in complex plotting in fiction. (Not all fiction is unpopular—violent and horror movies can be a particularly common

Box 3.4 Bodily movements

- Jumping with excitement.
- Unusual movements of hands and arms.
- Spinning self around.
- Rocking behaviour (sitting or standing up).
- Tip-toe walking.
- Aimless movement.

favourite in the autistic population—perhaps because they are so direct and emotionally stimulating).

Difficulties in describing emotions and feelings are also extremely common, in adults on the autism spectrum. The difference between the ability of neurotypical adults to describe their emotions in great detail, and the lack of that facility in someone on the autism spectrum, can be very striking. There is a growing literature on autism and *alexithymia*.[9] Such difficulties may also underlie the difficulty in seeing things from the perspective of others.

Bodily movements

In the intellectually disabled population it is common to observe in childhood and, sometimes, even into adulthood, a range of odd or unusual bodily movements. These are listed in Box 3.4. These bodily movements are rarely reported by observant informants of more able adults or are only described as having lingered on longer than expected in later childhood. Of these, the commonest unusual movement often observed in an adult is unusual stereotyped movement of hands or arms, which can also replace normal gesture.

Sensory differences

Interest in and recognition of the significance of differences in sensory experiences has grown in the past decade, possibly because there may be more scope to help affected individuals to cope with these characteristics, and with the growing voice of people writing and publishing their own accounts

---

[9] The inability to describe one's feelings, even in response to quite direct questions, should alert the clinician to ask is there a need to consider autism? See also the subheading 'Emotions' in Chapter 4, for a perspective of people on the autism spectrum.

of their experiences of autism (Grandin 2011). It has now entered an official list of criteria for autism, namely as set out in DSM-5 (American Psychiatric Association, 2013). However, as with many other descriptive features of the autism spectrum, we cannot yet be sure that it is confined to autism and that it does not occur in isolation in neurotypical individuals. A balanced summary overview of autism by a practicing neurologist makes interesting reading, which also refers to the concept of sensorimotor[10] abnormality (Rapin, 2011).

When sensory differences occur, is it important for it or for them to be recognized, given the potential significance for the person's needs in adjusting to different kinds of environments (as in 'reasonable adjustments', Chapter 13), which the affected person may not have control of, such as their work place and public spaces. Such differences may not be obvious to some observers such as family members and, in my view, can only be ascertained fully by an interview with the affected individual.

Sensory differences can be considered to occur in the form of decreased or increased sensitivity to the external world. Various forms of repetitive (increased) self-stimulation are inferred to be due to a state of under-stimulation. Being largely unaware of particular external stimuli, such as pain, and extremes of heat and cold, also suggest this kind of sensory difference, probably for different reasons. Heightened experience—or over sensitivity, appears to be more frequent, particularly in the more able adult. Sensory differences are also important because they are one of the areas in which it may be possible to take some steps to improve the quality of the lived experience of a child or adult on the autism spectrum (Chapter 13).

There may be some value in drawing a distinction between proximal and remote stimuli, as well as the more important, more widely recognized and described distinction between hyposensitivity and hypersensitivity, all forms of which can co-occur in the same individual. Before going on now to discuss examples of differences in sensitivity, it is also important to note that such sensory differences may change over time within the one individual.

Proximal (often repetitive) sensory stimuli

The behaviours listed in Box 3.5, appear to be rarely described in childhood or even later in the more able adult with autism. Those that do occur sometimes are repetitive touching of objects, tapping on surfaces, and non-injurious self-stimulation. Self-stimulation without injury raises the issue

---

[10] Relating to or involving both sensory and motor functions.

> **Box 3.5 Forms of proximal sensory stimulation (more likely to be encountered in the less able individual or in deprived, impoverished environments)**
>
> - Mouthing of objects.
> - Smelling objects or people.
> - Touching objects.
> - Scratching and tapping on surfaces.
> - Repetitive destructive activities.
> - Repetitive aimless manipulation of objects.
> - Self-injury.
> - Self-stimulation without injury.
> - Other forms of proximal sensory stimulation.

for clinicians of the threshold between self-stimulation and self-injury (Box 3.5). This is yet another alerting signal to the general psychiatric clinician to consider which or both of these categories such behaviour falls under.

As with so many experiences described as being associated with autism, such behaviours can be seen in isolation in many otherwise unaffected adults, for example, twiddling one's hair repetitively, rubbing one's beard, thumb sucking, carrying around and repeatedly touching a small, preferred object. Children also go through and then grow beyond normal stages of putting objects into the mouth, tasting, sniffing, etc.

Over sensitivity to sensory experiences

Although hearing is probably the most commonly affected sensory modality, all sensory modalities can be affected by over sensitivity.

Response to sounds Parents are often aware when their child is highly sensitive to certain sounds, to the point of experiencing pain. A useful distinction here may be made between acuity (ability to sense) and sensitivity (distress triggered by the sensation), which may require clinical interview probing and judgement. Many adults are (or used to be) very sensitive to the high pitched sound of a chalk stick being drawn across a blackboard, or to the sound of a creaking door. This pain and distress is what many persons on the autism spectrum describe in relation to a far wider variety of sounds that most other individuals hardly notice. These include, of course, loud and sudden sounds, but also certain mechanical sounds, such as electric pumps, hair dryers, the clicking of computer hard drive disks, and so forth. The sound of the human voice or of selected voices may also trigger discomfort and even pain. Sometimes there is heightened, but not distressing, sensitivity to certain sounds, so that the person can hear a sound long before other people they are with do so, such as the sound of an approaching train or other sound source.

Response to visual stimuli Geologists may be observed picking up and staring at objects from various angles, as may individuals on the autism spectrum, but in the latter case, with no purpose and no desire to share any noteworthy discoveries with others.

Box 3.6 lists examples of unusual responses to visual stimuli, most of which tend to have disappeared by adulthood.

Smell, taste, texture, temperature, pain Although already covered above, it is important to emphasize problems that can arise from over or under sensitivity to the sensory modalities of touch and smell, hot and cold temperature, and of pain. Occasionally, parents describe how their child fell and injured itself, but continued its activity, without telling a carer. One or two days later, when the child was observed to be walking in an odd way, or using an upper limb less than usual, further enquiry and a physical examination led to the diagnosis of a bone fracture. Over or under sensitivity to heat and cold could also have negative consequences for physical health.

Although this may not be important in all cases, it is very striking when a child or adult expresses very strict food preferences due to sensitivity to particular food textures. Choice of clothing may also be affected by an aversion to or a strong liking for a particular type of fabric, or for loose or for tight fitting clothing, both of which may result in a preference to wear the exact same clothing throughout the year, in all circumstances and in all climates.

Box 3.6 Response to visual stimuli

- Bright lights, shiny objects.
- Watching things spin.
- Twisting or turning hands or objects near the eyes.
- Interest in studying angles or objects.

Routines, repetitive behaviours, and resistance to change

Rigidity, repetitive behaviours, preference for sameness, dislike of novelty, a narrow and perseverative behavioural repertoire, circumscribed interests (fascinations), are also even more prominent than before in current classification rules. As with the topic of sensory difference, this is an area where the individual can describe and account for themselves at an interview. Carers will be aware of these traits and characteristics, although may not know how extensive they are or, indeed, any underlying emotional functioning.

There seems to be no satisfactory explanation as to why routines and resistance to change and sensory differences so often occur together in one individual. Furthermore, under the recent 5th revision of the DSM (American Psychiatric Association, 2013), they are grouped together.

From the point of view of adult psychiatry, there are three points of interest to make about these behaviours or differences. First, crucial to our work is the distinction from obsessive compulsive behaviours and ruminations. Outwardly it may be difficult to determine whether a behaviour that is repeated, is a sign of obsessive compulsive disorder or a pointer to autism. It may be difficult to make the distinction without asking the patient.

Fascinations and obsessions

Obsessional phenomena, as we know in psychiatry, are ego-dystonic, being perceived as against conscious resistance. Routines, rituals, and repetitive behaviours, observed in autism, are not ego-dystonic. Indeed, they are often perceived as pleasant and calming, as a way to 'unwind' at the end of a busy and stressful day. Lorna Wing used the word fascinations to make this crucial distinction from obsessions, which she said they are not. These distinctions would not matter were it not for their importance in management, because the autistic person with repetitive behaviours usually does not wish to relinquish them, but the patient with OCD would willingly do so. This distinction may not be 'hard wired': differences in the *substantia nigra* have been implicated in both (Bodfish, 2011).

Adaptive or disabling repetitive behaviours

The second point is that we think of autism as a neurodevelopmental disorder in which there is delay in many aspects of the normal development of behaviours that are adaptive and normal at some stage in early childhood. Repetitive behaviours, routines, and resistance to change are recognized as normal at the very early stages of development, but not later. They may have a role in learning early in development.

> **Box 3.7 Routines and resistance to change**
>
> - Clinging to home or familiar places.
> - Clinging to objects.
> - Collecting objects.
> - Arranging objects.
> - Maintenance of sameness of environment.
> - Maintenance of sameness in routines.
> - Acting out roles.
> - Circumscribed, narrow interests.
> - Collecting facts on specific subjects.
> - Activities related to special skills.

The third point is that all these behaviours can be observed in a mild and non-intrusive form in individuals who would not meet the criteria for autism. The extent to which such behaviour interferes with functioning is crucial to judging its clinical significance.[11] In the milder form, such 'traits' are not uncommon in families in which there is one individual with an autism diagnosis. Sometimes life is easier if one sticks to routines, and follows set patterns of behaving.

The range of routines and modes of resistance to change

A list of such behaviours is set out in Box 3.7 and is not exhaustive.

There are a number of reasons for an autistic adult to cling to home. Often it is that the social rules and expectations of the world outside are too difficult to tolerate. Sometimes it can be traced to a preference for familiarity and sameness, with no surprises and nothing unplanned. Adults have told the author that dealing with change takes so much energy and effort if called upon. Planning does not always work, but when it does it makes life much easier.

Clinging to and collecting objects becomes a problem when it develops into a level of hoarding behaviour that makes life impossible for others who share the same dwelling, if not for the hoarder. A specific distinction

---

[11] As DSM-5 was in development, insisting on this requirement reportedly resulted in a clash with the basic principle in DSM-5 that interference with functioning is a separately described requirement.

in autism is that collecting has no value or purpose, and there is no wish to share it with others. These are sometimes termed circumscribed interests. The collector of the memorabilia of a much loved football club is not interested in going to club matches with others who share the same interest. The precipitation of a sudden outburst of anger, when an object in one's surroundings is moved, may also be a problem. In childhood, parents often find ways of smoothing over this tendency (see Case Study B). In adulthood, it may undermine cohabitation and add further to social isolation.

Certain sensations, such as sounds or visual patterns, may also be a source of fascination and repetitive behaviour, including in our era the collection of audio files on a particular subject, such as the sounds of a particular breed of animal or bird. (These are harmless unless they take up so much time that essential day-to-day obligations are neglected). These should not be classed as sensory sensitivities (unless there is an element of distress). They are more likely to be about focal interests such as collecting. Some collecting may also represent a heightened sense of and fascination with visual or other patterns.

Routines can make life easier, especially as we grow older. Rigid insistence on routine, on the other hand, can drive others away. Interruptions in routine, for example, festivals, holidays, novel events, are often dreaded by children and adults on the spectrum who have this characteristic. It is not unusual for a patient given a clinic appointment for a set time to get up and leave the waiting room if the doctor or psychologist is not ready to see them, almost precisely on time. Similarly, if the patient's arrival is delayed due to heavy traffic, unreliable public transportation, or a problem in finding parking, they may give up and return home.[12]

Collecting objects and facts, and special interests, are a widely recognized feature of autism. They are common, but they are not essential in making the diagnosis. They are regarded as clinically significant when they impede other areas of activity that are necessary for independent living and occupation.

Routines and rituals

A *routine* is a sequence of actions regularly followed in the same particular order—examples are getting dressed in a set sequence, checking all the switches are off and windows are locked, before settling down at night, or systematically showering or bathing. While routines are, in themselves, a normal characteristic they become abnormal when unduly frequent, wasteful of time, or interfere with other activities.

A *ritual* consists of a series of actions that hold some additional, special significance for the person following them. Examples are an unusually

---

[12] Impatience may be a pointer to possible ADHD.

elaborate way of brushing teeth or grooming a dog, an unnecessarily complicated sequence for preparing or eating a meal, an unvarying sequence of phrases in opening a meeting as its chairman. As mentioned above, in autism, such behaviours are followed by choice and not against conscious resistance.

Behaviour problems in childhood and adulthood

The developing autistic child can also exhibit behaviours that are unusually challenging, with extreme expression of anger being a particular characteristic, and placing a great burden on the family. Such behaviour may lead to behaviours that place others outside the family at risk in later teen years and adulthood, but we do not yet know whether the overall amount of risk behaviour is different from that observed in the rest of the adult population.

Autism brings an increased risk of epilepsy and this may not emerge until the late teens. It may also be overlooked or over-shadowed because of an understandable tendency to attribute any unusual behaviour to an earlier diagnosis of autism. Most would agree that the developing brain in someone with autism is different and perhaps this is linked to the increased risk of epilepsy in autism recently confirmed to apply to general population and not just clinically ascertained subpopulations (Rai et al. 2012).

General (non-autistic) developmental characteristics important to a complete assessment

Studies of children with a diagnosis on the autism spectrum, followed-up into adulthood, show that possibly the most important predictor of a good outcome and independence in the community is general ability. Childhood IQ has consistently proved to be a reliable predictor of cognitive functioning well into mid- to- later adulthood (Howlin et al. 2014). Assessment of IQ is not covered here, but emotional development, motor development, self-care skills, independence, and academic performance (learning ability) play a major part in general developmental ability and should be considered as vital to the context in which autism is understood, although not a component part of the diagnosis. In Chapter 11, some of these will be discussed further under the heading of detailed needs assessment, making the distinction between cognitive, functional, motor, and emotional development.

Motor development

A common finding in the autism population is problems with gross motor co-ordination, described by carers as unusual clumsiness, which may include an impaired internal sense of the relative position of parts of one's

> **Box 3.8 General developmental indicators**
>
> - Language development (method of communication), understanding.
> - Motor co-ordination and large movements.
> - Fine movements and visuospatial skills.
> - Self-care skills.
> - School and academic work.
> - Independence.

own body (proprioception impairment). Occasionally, adults who only have such gross motor developmental problems, request an autism assessment although they rarely meet the criteria for autism. However, they may meet the criteria for Developmental Coordination Disorder (DCD) (American Psychiatric Association, 2013; see Chapter 10).

Box 3.8 provides a list of these developmental indicators. Some of these are particularly important in developing independence in adulthood, notably difficulties in attending to self-care.

Concluding points

In later chapters on assessment, and on support and care following diagnosis, the information in this chapter will be important in setting out what are the defining characteristics of autism. They also help us to appreciate how in the absence of 'magic bullet'[13] treatments, care, and support depends on recognizing, accepting, and working with them, both as the person with autism and as their doctor or psychiatrist, carer, companion, work supervisor, neighbour, or fellow citizen.

---

[13] The term 'magic bullet' is ambiguous as it may refer to a term coined during the pre-chemotherapy era, referring to what have since become the most powerful tools in medicine (e.g. antibiotics), or it could refer to unscrupulous researchers whose only goal is personal academic ambition and gain.

Chapter 4

Autism as a lived experience

A quote ...

'... [Oliver Sacks] learned about the importance of personal narrative for defining a meaningful life; this realization became central to both his clinical and literary practices. In 'The Anthropologist on Mars', an essay about Temple Grandin, a professor of animal behaviour who has autism, he defined a foundational principle for his 'existential neurology': 'while a single glance may suffice for clinical diagnosis, if we hope to understand the autistic individual, nothing less than a total biography will do'.[1]

Introduction

Those of us with experience of listening to adults, who come to our clinics with a request for an autism assessment, can provide numerous examples of the accounts of the *lived experience* of people who, we agree, have autism or significant autistic traits. A growing number of articulate adults, who are on the autism spectrum, have also written personal accounts of their experiences, covering their lives since diagnosis and also going back to childhood. These accounts have been helpful to us in developing questions to ask adults who are seeking an assessment, which bring out the core features of the condition, as they experience it. This chapter is very much about the perspective of people who we do find to have autism. Of course, at least some who come to such a diagnostic clinic, and who think they have autism (or the often preferred term 'Asperger syndrome'), do not have autism, but we will turn to that and how to differentiate these in Part II on assessment, mainly in Chapter 8.

The first part of this chapter takes us into issues that arise at the beginning of an assessment. The second part considers how people on the spectrum

---

[1] Reproduced from *Lancet*, 387(10021), Ann Jurecic, Daniel Marchalik, The literary legacy of Oliver Sacks, pp.835, Copyright 2016, with permission from Elsevier.

tend to describe their perspective on what we would view as the most striking signs of the presentation of autism, in terms of development since childhood, problems in communication and social adaptation, and a preference for order and predictability. Training courses on adult autism usually include such a personal account presented by an affected adult.[2]

Sources, including the self-diagnosed

There are no attributable case studies here and no verbatim quotes (unless clearly stated as such). Rather, what follows is akin to a qualitative synthesis of the common themes that patients with autism bring up again and again. However, this is not to claim that this is a formal qualitative data synthesis. Rather, it is a collection of repeated concerns and experiences of patients drawn from years of listening to them and to what their carers report they often say to them about their lives.

In preparing this chapter online, open chat rooms have also been accessed, such as the excellent and very responsibly (i.e. safely) maintained, discussion forum operated by the UK based National Autistic Society (http://community.autism.org.uk/discussions). The decision to do so was partly based on the importance of considering the perspectives of people who are less likely to come to a diagnostic clinic (we know most adults with autism have not done so).

It is important to point out that not everything written by people introducing themselves as having autism (or having one of its alternative titles, Asperger syndrome, high functioning autism, etc.), is any different from other self-reflective writing. Some is intended to be and a good deal succeeds helpfully in doing so.

In this chapter, material is highlighted that is more likely to be helpful in revealing the special perspective of those on the autism spectrum. The reader should not be biased into thinking that everything that is written down or claimed to be autism writing is what it claims to be. This will be important when we look at assessment techniques. Assessment techniques, contributions to chat rooms and discussion forums, as in the real world, sometimes also come from people who are not on the autism spectrum, although in some cases they may suggest that they are or genuinely believe that they are. Part of our role is to help some people to recognize that they may have strayed onto a different route and might benefit from considering a different set of explanations and solutions.

---

[2] A presentation by a carer of an adult with a late diagnosis can also add to the learning experience.

Perspective taking

As we know, a core feature of autism is a noticeable difficulty in seeing the world from the perspective of others. The perspective of someone with autism is often labelled 'egocentric' and it can certainly appear that way. (This is not a good term because often people on the autism spectrum struggle with a sense of self-identity.) In order to understand autism, to be more aware of it, and in order to help those affected, we too need to learn to be able to see their world as they see it. The best way to do this is to take the time to listen to their accounts of how they see the world and their attempts to deal with it.

The more we are asked to see older adults, who no longer have living parents who can describe their childhood, and current behaviour and functioning, the more important it is to have effective ways of drawing out the key pieces of information that could further such assessments. We also need to understand and accept how they see the world differently in order to help them have a good quality of life within a world that often seems quite irrational and even alien to them. The phrase 'I feel like a visitor from another planet—an "alien"—I don't feel I belong here', is frequently heard.

One of the purposes of this chapter is to help us build up the picture of the world experienced by adults on the spectrum, in order to suggest questions that could be useful in clinical practice, particularly where the patient is the only person available to us to provide the information needed to undertake an assessment (see Chapter 8) and in order to design effective coping mechanisms for the rest of their lives, in a sometimes alien world. To do this we also need to be able to take their perspective. Any training in clinical proficiency with autism must include time immersed in discussions, which are directed or, indeed, dominated by the contributions of people with the condition, and who are comfortable with and willing to talk openly about it. It can be like learning a new language requiring a period of immersion during which we allow our own prior perspective to be subordinated to the autistic perspective. The direct contribution of people with autism is an essential component of all training courses on autism designed for professionals. Most of us can probably imagine what it is like to be anxious, or depressed, or overwhelmed and paralysed into indecision. Seeing the world from an autistic perspective is, for most people, likely to be more difficult and, in training professionals, sometimes frustratingly difficult to achieve, although some will take to it with gratifying ease.

Self-expression—the challenge of getting started

Later in this chapter we will look at difficulties in communication from the perspective of the person with autism, but here it is useful to cover a few points that will arise as soon as an interview with a patient (who has autism) begins. Since the patient's perspective on the world is very different, (s)he may have few opportunities to talk about it. Encouraging someone, who we later establish has autism, to begin to talk about themselves can, for them, seem very difficult at first, although they will often say they have put enormous time into preparing for their first consultation. Anxiety or arousal levels may be unusually high—patients often describe feeling the need to refer to prepared notes, and are 'tongue tied'. As clinicians, we sometimes forget how daunting a first meeting with a psychiatrist can be; this may be even more challenging for the socially impaired adult. During the consultation, some ignore anything that is said, other than a quite specific direct question (and the risk is that direct questions can be leading and divert from the most important issues to be considered). Paradoxically, when patients do eventually begin to talk, they can soon switch into a speech-like monologue that is difficult to interrupt or halt, and may seem rambling.[3] (Often they are also quite self-conscious about how much they are digressing and 'wasting [your] time'.)

Being autistic means being slow to notice non-verbal cues from another person [i.e. from you the doctor] that signal to them [the patient], 'it's my turn to say or ask something now'. It is as if they have been silently building up in their minds a long and very detailed account of their lives, which is suddenly released. Some on the autism spectrum refer to this using the computer analogy of a 'data dump' (there is no humorous intent here). Attempts to interrupt this flow can produce irritated reactions. This is not anger (although expressions of anger can occur suddenly). A common complaint of people on the autism spectrum is that interruptions are hugely problematic—in more extreme cases the only way to resume is to start over again at the beginning. Equally, they are sometimes aware of this. 'I know I talk on too much, but I just don't know when to stop, the way other people seem to know with its time to give way'.

Although we often think of people on the autism spectrum as saying very little, this does not mean that they have nothing to say. Observations of this kind will be covered in more detail in Chapter 9.

---

[3] Distractibility and 'mind wandering' could be an alerting signal to ADHD.

Making a difference—for example, staying in employment—making adaptations to the perspective of the adult with autism

People who have received their diagnosis on the autism spectrum as adults often describe the striking difference diagnosis makes to their lives.[4] Before diagnosis life is difficult and puzzling. Once diagnosed, and once an opportunity has been provided to learn with others about how the two worlds differ, the autistic and the neurotypical, it becomes possible to make more sense, or at least to navigate through the world, while still being who you are.

Having autism can mean feeling (and being) excluded in many ways that require natural social ability. Let us take employment as an example. It is not surprising that many affected adults describe finding rule-based employment easier and, therefore, more rewarding (working in a warehouse, in the store room of a food shop, or in the part of a library that customers do not access, are all less stressful because it is so much easier to follow a very strict and detailed rule-based structure).

Contrast this with working with customers and the public (at the customer counter, or the till), which are far more difficult and stressful. To the person affected by autism, all the expectations of other people in such settings seem 'pointless' (although to us 'friendly'), such as the things that customers say, for example, about 'the weather' or 'the traffic' (neither of which, from the perspective of the person with autism, 'you can do anything about—so why mention them?') For example, if such a staff member is asked by a customer to point out where a particular item is, e.g. on a shelf in the shop, the customer will be led noticeably quickly to precisely the right place. Alternatively, the customer may be told, again very precisely and perhaps abruptly—'the last one sold this morning at 11:15'. There may be no word of apology. Being polite is not wired in—appearing to be impolite is not intended.

Making autism visible to the person with the condition and key others can create a crucial bridge out of this isolation so that training can be provided to adjust for such difficulties in a particular context. Through training of such employees, a lack of intuitive sympathy may be replaced by learned manners. Training to show sympathy is feasible, although without training it may come through conscious deduction by a particularly capable individual on the autism spectrum. More often than not, explicit training may be the only solution for an employer that values employees with such reliable

---

[4] An insistence on a clear 'yes' or 'no' reply to the question 'am I autistic?' can also be an issue that requires discussion, given the dimensional nature of autism.

and responsible attention to detail. It may be possible, with training and experience, to get used to such settings, provided the perspective of the staff member is appreciated and understood.

The accounts of adults on the autism spectrum also include the experience of having adapted to work settings in which their difficulties were not accommodated, and in which they had to go to great efforts to 'fit in'. Sometimes it goes well. For example, colleagues notice that the person is 'very good at solving detailed technical problems, adapting to new technologies' and so the person becomes highly valued (even though in no way qualified for such new responsibilities). On the negative side, success eventually brings closer the day when promotion to a more managerial role, with all the social communication skills that requires, creates its own difficulties and stresses. Similarly, the more time spent settled into a job, the sooner or later the job is changed or reorganized, with changed routines and timetables, which may prove so stressful that the person may quit the job. Sometimes this can mean avoiding any further employment experience, social isolation, and a dramatic reduction in income.

Alternatively, stress may lead to taking time off work. Disciplinary reviews may arise due to misunderstandings and complaints by subordinates, which the person finds difficult to comprehend (i.e. 'everything makes no sense', 'is illogical'). The person may not realize that they should seek to be represented (and representatives, such as union officials, may completely fail to recognize the person's needs). It is only when autism is recognized as a disability that, with the benefit of hindsight, the difficulties begin to make sense. There are positive accounts of understanding and appreciative bosses, managers, who make a huge difference for the affected person's working life.

The importance of employment and of making reasonable adjustments, and other effective actions will come up again in Chapters 13 and 14.

Return on investment—keeping carers on board

Some patients have remarked on how they first found their way to a diagnostic clinic. At the time they attend, they may be very unclear as to why this has been suggested. They go along with the suggestion because of a carer, usually a parent, but also partners in the case of older adults. When asked why they have come there will usually be a pause. The person with autism may seem to struggle with a reason for being there. There are occasions when they are in the clinic because they have been left with little choice but to be there. In Chapters 5 and 6, the important topic of why adults decide to seek a diagnosis [or not to] will be expanded upon.

Two explanations seen sometimes can be attributed to carers bringing about the initiation of an assessment. This may arise when the carer is close to giving up and to abandoning the person they have been trying to care for. A parent may be deeply concerned as to whether their adult offspring will ever manage to cope independently when they are no longer there. In desperation, carers will do anything to find understanding and recognition in the health and care system.

The second explanation, which can be much difficult to manage professionally, is where the patient is coming because a long-term partner has left them with little choice in the matter. A diagnosis of autism has become the last possible explanation for a crumbling relationship (relationship breakdown and living outside a stable relationship are clearly associated with autism in the general population, including among the large number of relatively mildly affected cases). The doctor may be their last chance. Often they both need help as individuals in their own right, probably before they try to engage in couple advice or counselling.

Making sense of it all—'it has to make sense or it doesn't make sense!'

The majority may have worked out a reason for asking or at least acceding to an assessment. The argument (which someone else may have suggested first), which often makes most sense, is that knowing if autism is an explanation gives them a reason, something to work with. Knowing the cause may make it possible to resolve some of the issues they live with. Sometimes that simple hope seems touching and naive. It may be a good point at which to start a positive process.

A medical explanation may also make their difficulties more acceptable to others, instead of being viewed as unsociable or difficult. Some may refer, albeit somewhat vaguely, to the hope that if there is a reason, others may be more tolerant and perhaps even helpful. Getting a sick note from the doctor, for example, may be less stressful once a diagnosis has been made official. Rather concrete analogies to computer and data technology are often used. One can think of this as the 'engineer's view of the world' (i.e. if you know what is broken you can mend it—it's just a problem to be solved, like anything else). Patients requesting an assessment may also think or even refer to resources in the community that could help them.

A journey that began in childhood or that had no beginning

The adult with autism (until now undiagnosed) will very often look back on an unhappy childhood (or so it seems—they are unlikely to put it that way—having little facility for describing emotions and feelings at any time).

Experiences of having been bullied are so ubiquitous that an absence of such a history should cause us to question whether the person is autistic, particularly in the case of males. They may underplay its importance. Sometimes they will have told a parent who may have intervened—or an older (or rarely younger) sibling who 'fixes it' in a way they could not.

When asked about making friends as a child there may be another blank pause. Without quite a lot of more specific probes (Chapter 8), it may be difficult to get an account. Birthday parties will have been unhappy occasions that 'you had to put up with'. Some will recognize the effort put in by a parent to normalize their relationships with their peers, albeit to little avail. The happy (or better 'stress-free') times of childhood will, more likely, have been the times spent alone with video, electronic games, constructional toys, etc. It may have included playing football—but questions about how else time was spent around football will often draw another blank. Peers may also have led them into difficulties with authority figures that made little or no sense, such as being led into behaviour that is antisocial without being able to anticipate the consequences and often being the kid who gets caught when the others have made off.

Two-way interaction: communication and 'un-communication'

Two-way interaction is often described as only possible with one other person at a time. Knowing how and when to join in with any more than one other person is an endless puzzle. Informality is viewed as 'pointless', 'bizarre', and worst of all, 'misleading'. Dealing in straight facts is greatly preferred, only in as much as it is necessary.

Chit chat—'what's that?'

One of the things many patients have quite spontaneously said is that it is impossible to talk unless there is 'something to talk about'. Therefore, talking about themselves is not so difficult (adults on the autism spectrum can make great spokespersons and lecturers on the topic of autism). The more observant adult on the autism spectrum, having tried to engage in socialization and largely given up on it, will complain critically that we 'neurotypicals' (i.e. us) 'waste so much time *talking about nothing*'. (We call this conversation, 'chit chat'). For example, 'the weather'—'you neurotypicals say such rubbish about weather! Why don't you just check the meteorology forecast in the morning and shut up about it!' 'What's the point' about saying 'oh it's a nice day, today', or 'I wish we could see an end to this cold damp weather', when the answer is in the meteorology forecast and there's 'nothing to talk about!'

As we shall see later, any assessment does need to include a form of testing to check out whether the patient is able to 'talk about nothing'—in a social way. The direct Q&A style we are all trained to follow in medicine, is much easier for the autistic patient to follow. Suddenly being expected to be chatty is much more challenging. This distinction is crucial to good and effective clinical practice because autism may be missed unless the consultation includes the challenge that comes with shifting unexpectedly to a conversational style.[5]

Taking it literally and needing clarity

Adults on the spectrum often remark that the way other people behave 'does not make sense', 'is irrational'. We (neurotypicals) are accused of being 'inconsistent', 'don't mean what they [you] say', 'don't say what they [you] mean' and consequently are 'impossible to deal with'. 'You say one thing but you mean another'. With time they may learn to work out what we really mean, but doing so can be exhausting. 'You said you would call at 10.00 a.m.' 'But you never arrive on time'. 'Why say so if you don't mean it?' 'I arrive on time and you turn up late'. 'That messes me up for the day'. 'It can take hours to settle down again'.

Reasonable explanations (often provided by a patient's carer), are quickly dismissed (distress is more likely conveyed clearly through such direct encounters and less adequately communicated in conventional enquiries we might use).

Preferences in communication

Some modes of communication are far easier than others. Group discussion is usually the most challenging. There is much current public concern about our reliance on communication by text (on a smartphone) interrupting 'real contact' between people. However, if you are on the spectrum, the former (text) may be your most favoured mode of communication with others, including your peers. A preference for communication through text can be seen in the preference for online technology as a means for making contact

---

[5] One of the paradoxes of our often rule-driven world is that the narrative style expected in a book such as this is formal and dry, but nowadays, teaching the same material, in person, in a group, brings with it an expectation of informality and a conversational style that might not suit every learner.

and, occasionally, enabling meeting others, playing (as in online computer games), and avoiding 'pointless chit chat and conversation'. It seems that online you 'have to have something to communicate about'.[6]

Autistic preference for communicating with work associates has also crept into the 'typical' world. In many work settings we tend increasingly to use email, rather than to meet and talk, but for the person on the spectrum the clarity and the value of the written record to refer back to and to avoid misunderstanding is a huge advantage.

Social functioning

The social world is the single greatest challenge. 'It doesn't make sense'. 'Others seem to get on fine. Why not me?' Joining in is 'demanding and exhausting'. Avoiding contact is easier but can be lonely. 'I have always been different, an outsider', etc.

What a friend is (not)

Friendship is widely recognized to be an area of substantial difficulty. Friendship is viewed quite differently. There is a need for clear rules in a world in which there are very few written rules about friendship. However, the first mistake clinicians often make, who have not thoroughly embraced the topic of autism, is in thinking that if a patient says 'I have friends', that rules out autism. People with autism have a different perspective on friends. Again, there must be purpose for contact with others. In the same way as having to talk and chat 'about nothing' is off-putting, being with a friend must have 'some purpose'. Being able to share a game or an intellectual challenge makes contact worthwhile. It is often painfully hard to make sense of relationships. 'Why did (s)he suddenly drop me?' When friendships break down (a boy/girl friend stops calling or phoning up or dating) there can be puzzlement, considerable distress, and not unusually a firm and unshakable decision to 'never get involved in that way again'. Often 'aspies' find the company of other 'aspies' more congenial. Parents may remark that their offspring often seemed drawn to other kids who are vulnerable.

Chilling out—'company isn't everything its claimed to be'

Time enjoyed being active, alone, has all sorts of merits. 'You have control'. 'You can spend as much time engaged in activity on your own as you choose'. 'You

---

[6] Apparently, some online chat lines are 'closed'—that is, they are only open to persons who can make a convincing case that they are on the autism spectrum.

can chose to deal with ordered parts of the world'—computers, rule-based systems, such as games, collecting information, collecting objects that fall into a particular category. 'Chilling out' is a time to 'recharge the battery', needed to face the world of people, including carers. However, this may only be safe and comfortable if you have a family or someone to fall back on, who is watching out for you.

Public misunderstanding

Carers will be concerned that their son or daughter is not aware of how others view them in public, not to mind at a job interview, or at a visit to an employment centre. This can be a major source of stress for parents of a growing child, because of their behaviour in public and their lack of understanding of social rules.[7] Adults on the spectrum find that dealing with strangers, the public, work, school and college can give rise to stressful social misunderstandings. If a person is autistic it is not always clear to them what the rules of social engagement are. 'You can't ask anyone what the rules are' because they will 'look at you as if you are just crazy'. Questions that may pose a huge challenge include 'how do you ask a girl for a date?' How do you say 'yes' to a boy who wants to 'go out with you' (and what does 'going out' mean?), and similar problems to be faced for the first time, 'without having to fight free of being assaulted, or raped'. Even when there seem to be written instructions, and rules, they can be illogical, misleading, totally lacking in clarity.[8]

Having a recognized diagnosis can change these difficulties for the better—it should mean having someone you can ask—and knowing where to look for information in written or in video form (Chapters 12 and 13).

Emotions

Remarkably often, adults on the autism spectrum, when asked to describe feelings and emotions, struggle to do so. Emotions that are described are: anger (known as 'rants', 'meltdowns'), anxiety ('panics'), perplexity, 'information overload', 'too much'. Strategies for avoiding such states are often based on advance planning and preparation. (As mentioned earlier,

---

[7] Blurting out something quite inappropriate could equally be a sign of ADHD (see Chapter 10).

[8] The development of online social networking and other online resources is changing how young people on the autism spectrum are trying to solve such problems, which we also need to be aware of.

the consultation is often one of those events that create anticipatory anxiety, and planning may include visiting the clinic building, before the appointed date, just to be sure where it is and how you get in.) Patients who have experienced pathological anxiety or depression will often be better able to describe these emotions.

A key point for clinicians is that it is unsafe to assume that autistic patients' descriptions of emotions correspond to those of typical patients. We will come to this in considering the assessment of comorbidity (Chapter 10).

Independence—'making do'

Problems with surviving—paying bills, managing paperwork—will form a major part of any discussion. Even seemingly able adults, including university graduates, may struggle far longer than expected to develop these basic skills of independence. They will describe, if asked, spending money on purchases that they do not need, and going hungry or unable to pay the rent as a consequence. When this becomes repeatedly painful and stressful (especially having to cope with debt), they may begin to plan and think methodically. The advent of online banking has been a huge step forward for the more able adult on the spectrum, because they can set up automatic billing systems.

Many younger adults on the autism spectrum, who are continuing to live with and to depend on parents, often show a striking indifference to their dependency on carers and to the little that they contribute towards or share in the responsibilities of running a home. Carers will say that their son or daughter will only help if asked to. The individual when asked will acknowledge that sometimes they 'only empty the dishwasher', for example, 'when reminded to'. Parents sometimes do not seem to realize that quite often, once their offspring is living independently, they will very quickly take responsibility for such routine tasks. However, occasionally additional support will be needed at such times. This point is taken up further below.

Adults on the spectrum sometimes present in odd or unusual clothing—either very striking and conspicuous (see Case Study C, 2), or very bland and drab. It may surprise you to find how much care and thought has been put into these choices. It will seem highly egocentric—lacking in consideration of how it is viewed by others. It may be very functional. There is an impression that women on the spectrum often try to imitate, in what they wear, a revered figure such as a celebrity (although not appreciating that what they are imitating is costume, rather than day-to-day behaviour). Indeed, some look as if they are dressing up for a public performance. Knowing who their preferred celebrity is may help trigger an opening up of conversation and discussion, although preoccupations and fascinations such as these can take over a consultation, if one is not careful.

Sensory differences and experiences

The contribution of people with autism to our understanding of their perspective is most strikingly illustrated by the growing understanding and knowledge of the importance of sensory differences in autism, which they have given to us. For Temple Grandin, this is one of her two top priorities for research to help people with autism (Grandin, 2011): 'sensitivity to noise, fluorescent lights, scratchy clothes, or strong smells is a serious problem for many individuals with autism and Asperger's syndrome'. She points out the irony that the number of research studies on theory of mind outnumbers the number on sensory problems over a hundred times, arguing that 'normal people have a huge deficit in sensory theory of mind'. She uses the term 'scrambling' to refer to the difficulty in screening out a distracting stimulus, particularly when it causes actual pain. This can lead to 'sensory overload' where it becomes impossible for the person to function. It can make the autistic person more reliant on sensory modalities that are not affected by trying to ignore or shield out those that are. If hearing is affected it may be possible to rely on touch and smell instead. This must appear very odd to others—hence, the importance of identifying such phenomena and making sense of them (and certainly not labelling them as psychotic). Taste sensitivity can explain seemingly rigid dietary restrictions (avoidances and preferences).

Preference for predictability and sameness

People on the autism spectrum can describe with little or no difficulty habits, predictability, clearly planning ahead, comfortable familiarity, fascinations—other than that they may not appreciate how others view such behaviours. People on the spectrum talk quite calmly and nonchalantly about their habits and rituals. For them, this is not a problem, although if it results in reckless expenditure, it will probably become a problem.

Problems begin when others place restrictions on these preferences and behaviours. They view as unwelcome and unwanted any suggestion that a treatment be taken to reduce such behaviours. Extremely common is the irritation, annoyance, even pain, caused by other people's unreliability, poor punctuality, etc.

A striking feature of so many of these preferred behaviours, including narrow interests, collections, and repetitive behaviours, is the absence of much if any inclination to share them with others. These so-called 'circumscribed interests' have no intrinsic purpose other than being for their own sake. The person on the spectrum, devoting time in this way, often seems a little puzzled when asked do they enjoy meeting others who have the same interest, although well organized opportunities for doing so are well advertised. If they have visited such settings, the experience has usually been unrewarding and sometimes even stressful.

Impact and 'missing out'

As mentioned above, it can be surprising how little thought has been given by the young adult on the spectrum to the impact of their behaviour on others, in regard to daily necessities and duties. One is struck, often, by how little awareness there seems to be about the level of reliance they are placing on carers. The cost, emotional and material, born by carers is often not appreciated until it is no longer there. There is something quite child-like[9] about this. Questions about these kinds of issues are also often responded to with a degree of puzzlement.

It is only when attempting to live independently that the effects of their way of seeing and interacting with the world has its costs for them. A lack of appreciation of responsibilities and duties may not capture their attention until it must do so of necessity. One sometimes sees in families how a younger sibling, recognizing this, steps in and provides understanding care and support. The cost in difficulties in relationship functioning can be particularly striking. Isolation and loneliness can play an enormous part. Neglect of physical health and poor personal hygiene, should also be considered, as other agencies may not have been able to recognize and monitor it.

A better future?

Although covered in Part III, it is worth pointing out here that there are big changes to the lives of adults on the spectrum following assessment and diagnosis (good and not so good). Importantly, instead of criticizing and blaming themselves for not being able to fit in, a different, opposite view emerges. With growing experience of adult life, it can become possible to 'learn how the world works'. It may also mean encountering the wider world less—'as little as necessary'—with some knowledge and experience of what the neurotypical world expects or demands, no matter how 'illogical and

---

[9] Child-like behaviour may also be an alert to possible mild intellectual disability (see Chapter 10).

pointless' it may seem to be. It can be very helpful, in reviewing the progress of a patient post-diagnosis, to spend part of the consultation with a carer present—their contributions and comments can efficiently reveal the distinction between the perspective of the one being supported from the wider world.

It is essential that information imparted is also provided in written and sometimes even in diagrammatic form. As may sometimes be the case, if too much information is being imparted that leads to 'information overload', the carer may be able to absorb some of the finer details and share them later with the patient.

How to approach the task of assessment should now be clearer. The care pathway from initial awareness (by patient and doctor), through to producing a diagnosis-led care plan should now make sense. We now have an underpinning structure of understanding of the nature of autism in adulthood, of how it differs from typical development and, finally, how it is perceived and viewed by the affected adult.

Part II

The Clinical Assessment and Diagnostic Pathway

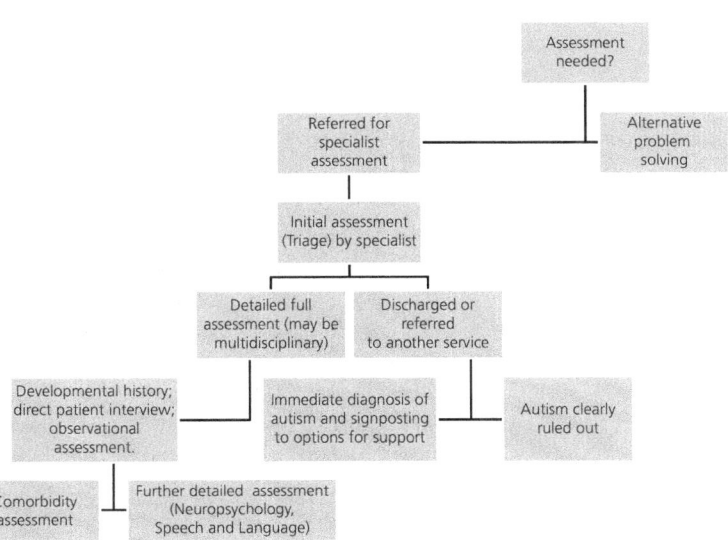

Fig. P.II Overview of the assessment process from referral through to diagnosis or discharge.

Chapter 5

Obtaining an assessment

Introduction

This book is written to help psychiatrists who see adults, to meet growing challenges and expectations on services to support people with autism. The main purpose of this chapter is to consider how to obtain an assessment by referring to a service that provides autism assessments. Referral to a specialist service may entail unacceptably long delays, which neither helps the patient nor assists in the efficient working of the service currently seeing him or her. An assessment provided by an appropriate specialist will be needed sometimes; it can also be an invaluable opportunity to learn more about the condition. Thus, this book may encourage and enable psychiatrists themselves to be able to learn to assess, diagnose, and where required, manage adults known to be on the autism spectrum. However, until sufficient experience (preferably if possible under supervision) and confidence is built up in diagnosing autism, there will continue to be times when an outside opinion and advice is needed, unless a diagnosis has already been clearly made.

Part II begins in this chapter with the process of obtaining an assessment, possibly the first step a clinician may seek, having become aware of the possibility of autism in a patient, but not being ready or confident enough to perform an assessment themselves. The remainder sets out the details of the assessment processes, divided into four parts (see Fig. P.II):

- Triage (checking whether a suspicion that an assessment is needed is correct, Chapter 6).
- Obtaining a developmental history (ideally from a parent with a good recollection of the patient's childhood as well as current functioning, Chapter 7).
- Interviewing the patient taking an approach that is quite like an assessment of psychopathology in an adult with an acute mental illness, but focusing on patterns across life since childhood (Chapter 8).

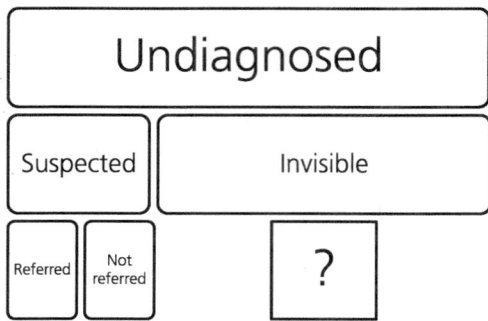

Fig. 5.1 Illustrative diagrammatic representation of the total population of adults with autism according to whether recognized, and whether or not referred for an assessment.

♦ Systematically approaching the description and evaluation of observed behaviour, particularly styles of communication and non-verbal interaction (Chapter 9).

Some elements of Part II (Chapters 6–11) may require specialist training and others will be more straightforward—much depending on whether the particular case is complex. The first (Chapter 6) covers the steps to be undertaken in an initial assessment designed to decide if a more detailed assessment is warranted.

Running throughout this chapter and the next, on initial (triage) assessments, is an ongoing consideration of the question of whether or not to recommend a detailed assessment and, if so, how detailed it needs to be. Our knowledge of the epidemiology of autism in adulthood suggests that most adults with the condition are unrecognized and undiagnosed (Brugha et al. 2011) (Fig. 5.1). We do not know this, but it is quite possible that many such undiagnosed adults cope quite well, other than during occasional life crises. Identification, if in later adulthood, might raise expectations of change and adjustment, which could be counterproductive in the longer term. Carers may have unrealistic expectations of change, although good and timely advice about autism should obviate this. The diagram illustrates the issues.

In adult clinical settings the psychiatrist is more likely to see patients, who have had an autism assessment at some point since childhood, compared with, for example, the patient seen in primary care settings.[1] We do not have

---

[1] This chapter may also be useful for the interested primary care physician, for whom Chapter 10 on comorbidities may also be important in deciding whether autism is the principle issue.

trial evidence to guide us on when a person will be better off knowing they have the condition. A decision to refer (or to initiate an assessment), will depend on a careful consideration of the trade-offs involved. Diagnosis may bring with it a label that is difficult to shake off and barriers to inclusion in society. Ignorance may result in unnecessary suffering and less effective measures to reduce its negative consequences, out of lack of the knowledge and experience that could help tackle its challenges and negative effects.

Role of specialist services in offering assessments

General psychiatrists are more likely to take on assessment responsibilities knowing that a specialist colleague, with whom they can consult, is close to hand; the same will be true for physicians working in primary care. However, there is a shortage of such specialist services for adults. This gap possibly derives from the lack of priority given to autism in general medical and psychiatric service development and in professional training. This shortage may also be due to such adults not seeking an explanation for their difficulties in the form of a medical diagnosis, so that demand is low. This is in clear contrast to the, generally better, health and educational service provision for autism in childhood, expected by parents and teachers. All of these factors will determine success in obtaining an assessment during adult life.

Any psychiatrist (or general practitioner, clinical psychologist or paediatrician) will know how difficult it can be to obtain an assessment for an adult they suspect of having autism. Specialist services are scarce and, in some areas, non-existent. Many have commented, most particularly parents, on the sudden gap in services when a child with known autism enters the adult age group (see Chapter 14). In a few countries, services are developing (see also Chapter 14) in recognition of the needs of the adult population.

A second issue is knowing what type of service is best equipped to help. And a third issue is the nature of the service, the skills and qualifications of the professionals. Funding mechanisms are also an issue in some geographic areas, particularly for the working age adult, who may not be eligible for financial support and who may have a poor income, employment record and no way of obtaining re-imbursement for costs.

Reasoned case for an assessment—making an effective referral

As demand grows, services increasingly expect referral requests to be well evidenced, with a clearly argued case for need. A referral of an adult is more likely to be considered and accepted by a well-regarded and busy autism service if a clear case of need can be made. Because autism is normally a life-long condition, there should be no need for an adult, who has had an autism diagnosis in childhood, to have their diagnosis re-evaluated in adulthood. There may be instances where due to improvements in skills or the loss of a care environment, for further assessment to be carried out. As early recognition grows, the need for diagnostic assessments in adulthood can be expected to decline.[2] Clearly records of an assessment in childhood must be checked before considering an assessment need any further.

The patient and often the person most closely involved in caring for them, such as a parent who is growing older, will be well placed to supply much of the necessary information needed in developing a case for referral of an adult who has not been assessed previously.

Could the need be met in other ways through simple problem solving?

Individual need may not always be best met through referral to a specialist service. Through epidemiological case finding studies, we continue to build up knowledge informing us of the characteristics of adults meeting criteria for autism, but who are, as yet, undiagnosed. Although the picture is still unclear, it is possible that there are many such individuals in the community who are leading reasonably acceptable independent lives. We already know that they do not seek mental health advice from health services in England in the way that a significant proportion of adults with other mental disorders do. (http://content.digital.nhs.uk/catalogue/PUB21748). There may be occasional crises in their lives, but given how long it can take to obtain an assessment, any quick decision to refer should not be made in someone who seems to have been settled for long periods of time.

One should ask what, if anything, each patient wants. Consider what unwanted impact the condition (if present) may have—and, if so, is there another more direct way of addressing it? The person may seem quite socially isolated, but do they prefer it to be like that? Can other changes be made that would help? What local resources such as groups or activities might meet the need that does not require a prior diagnosis? If the patient

---

[2] In some countries the identification in schools of need for childhood educational support can be judged by school learning support teachers. Therefore, the need for a medical diagnosis is removed. However, if exceptional or highly costly remedial services are required, more detailed educational psychology, paediatric, or child and adolescent psychiatry assessment may be justified.

suspected of autism is apparently having difficulties in a key setting, such as employment, marriage, independent living, can simple, but effective adjustments be made without needing to undertake a potentially elaborate and slow diagnostic process? Even if it were to prove later that autism was not relevant, simple problem-solving may be very welcome in its own right.

A useful lesson gained from studying 'alternative medicine' approaches to medicine, is the realization that so many people try alternatives of their own before turning to orthodox medicine. It behoves us to know what else our patients are or have been trying. Lydia Andal has published a book on self-diagnosis (Andal, 2015). This is a reminder that people will try to work out if they are affected by autism either without or, at least, before seeking an assessment. It includes a tip that several patients have followed, because they did not want their families to know they were having an assessment. They drew up a list of possible developmental differences described in autism (as in Chapter 3) and, over a series of conversations with parents, asked what each of the children (they and their siblings) in the family were like, in regard to each possible developmental difference. This was probably better than nothing, but it left one as a clinician somewhat in the dark, as one did not know if the parent understood each question and was replying reasonably accurately, or was engaging in exaggeration or denial. Nor did one know how selective their offspring was being in reporting back the answers they obtained from the family.

For the primary care physician, a recent publication on referral and alternatives to referral, by general practitioner (primary care physician), Dr Yasmin Delargy, can be strongly recommended (Delargy, 2013). This includes the valuable advice to the primary care physician to enter onto the patient record the suspicion, or preliminary view, that autism may be present and may need to be considered, in the event of a future unexpected crisis.[3] This might also be something to bear in mind if the patient, later in life, needed to go into hospital for medical reasons, where reasonable adjustments might need to be made and hospital staff briefed. The patient should, of course, be kept informed of any such steps.

Information needed to inform an assessment

Box 5.1 is a useful checklist of information to consider including in a referral.

Most clinics either require or make a strong point to the patient that they be accompanied to any assessment by a parent or suitable carer, or a

---

[3] A pilot evaluation of such a coding scheme, by PHCs/GPs was in process in early 2017, in England, funded from central government.

> **Box 5.1 Written information required for an adult autism assessment referral**
>
> - Has never been assessed for autism previously (e.g. in childhood).
> - Consents to being assessed and has the capacity to decide on the benefits and any risks.
> - Availability of a third party informant with lifelong knowledge of the adult.
> - Patient consents to involving an informant in the assessment process.
> - Patient reasons for seeking a referral and how it might help them.
> - Informant concerns and reasons for suspecting autism as an explanation.
> - Evidence of impact on functioning including ability to manage independently.
> - Relevant medical and psychiatric history, including psychiatric co-morbidity (Chapter 10 and Box 10.1 checklist), and treatment and relevant issues of risk.
> - Observations and judgement of need for assessment by referring physician.

long-term confidante; consent for such third party involvement should be sought and documented. Sometimes a long waiting time is needed for the patient to come around to recognizing the necessity for this. As we shall see in the following chapters, in Part II, a developmental history can be crucial in differentiating autism from another developmental or long-term form of mental disorder, with very important implications for advice and management.

It is recommended that an initial discussion take place, when a referral is being considered, with an agreement that the patient and or carer will draft reasons for seeking a diagnostic referral (Box 5.2). The reasons should include answers to such questions as: 'why I think I have autism (or 'Asperger syndrome'); in what way an assessment would help; how I understand myself and get things wrong; how it affects my life including work and earnings, ability to run a home or join with others in doing so, gain the most from education, pursue leisure activities at a place and time that is not distressing, have contact with companions and friend's so that I am not isolated and lonely'.

> **Box 5.2 Possible reasons for seeking a referral**
>
> - Why the patient thinks they have an autism spectrum disorder.
> - How it seems to affect my life.
> - Why an assessment could help.
> - Specific problems such as difficulties with living independently.
> - Difficulties in taking part in further training and education.
> - Isolation and loneliness, and holding onto friends.
> - Getting and keeping a job.

Because autism traits are widely spread throughout the population, specialist services are more likely to consider referrals that provide good information on significant impact on functioning and in some contexts impact and burden on others. There should also be included mentions of serious concerns and potential risks, such as of self-harm, vulnerability in the community and, although rare, possible risks to others. Risk assessments should be up to date because a specialist clinic may not be in a position to identify risks that are not part of the reason for an autism assessment itself.

It is important to consider whether a suspicion of autism is correct by considering common alternative explanations for long term and persistent relationship difficulties, including key comorbidities (Chapter 10, Box 10.1), attention deficit hyperactivity disorder (ADHD), other neurodevelopmental disorders, and adult personality disorder. Include the past history in particular of mental health issues, including treatments, and of other health problems. Include any records of assessments in childhood by paediatric, child psychiatry, or educational psychology services. Summarize behaviours that have been observed or reported suggestive of an autism spectrum disorder (ASD). Refer to diagnostic guidelines such as the International Classification of Diseases (ICD-10; World Health Organization, 1993)—an 11th version is due to be ratified and published officially in 2018), or the Diagnostic and Statistical Manual of the American Psychiatric Association (American Psychiatric Association, 2013). Describe whether there are concerns about risk. Indicate how often the patient seeks support—through unusually frequent consultation.

The referral could helpfully include information based on direct observation of the patient in the practice consultation setting (Box 5.3). (It would be helpful also to be able to describe the patient's behaviour in other less structured settings, such as in a waiting area or, if observed, in the local

> **Box 5.3 Observational information to include in a referral**
>
> - Behaviour observed in one or more setting by referring physician or colleagues including administrative staff.
> - Interaction with other people in informal settings, such as waiting areas.
> - Use of gesture, eye gaze, facial expression, vocal intonation.
> - Form of response to questions (brief, extended; concrete, informal, formal).
> - Restlessness and anxiety.

community, or within the patient's home during a home-based consultation). How does the patient interact in the setting? Does (s)he engage using appropriate eye gaze, gesture, variation in facial expression. Is speech over-formal, elaborate, drifting into irrelevance? Are responses to questions brief and monosyllabic, over-concrete, and are there any responses to comments made by the doctor? For further details see Chapter 9.

Patients may exhibit certain behaviours that indicate the severity of their difficulties. For example, a patient may be reluctant to attend and wait in a consultation waiting area (it is good practice to offer to arrange for the patient to be allowed to wait outside the clinic, for example, in a car or at a nearby cafe, and to be sent an electronic text message shortly before the doctor is ready to see them).

Evaluating and using tests for informing a referral

In many other areas of medicine and psychiatry tests are available to referring doctors that specialist services often find helpful in assisting with a decision to make a referral. Before discussing the available tests in this area, a few points need to be made as to how to determine whether a test is cost effective (McNamee 2003).

Clearly users of the test must be able to complete it unaided or with the support of an adult who does not behave in a way that may bias the result. Given that autism is associated with reduced IQ, this will preclude the use of a written, self-completion test in cases in which the patient lacks adequate reading ability. Tests are sensitive to differences between populations partly due to variations in the frequency of occurrence of the condition. Thus, a test that works well in one setting, such as with university undergraduate students, may not in a different setting, such as a primary care clinic serving an urban industrial community. A test may produce misleading results if it has not been evaluated for the purpose for which it is needed in the population from which the patient is drawn. Specialist services may refuse to consider a referral based on a test that they have found produces large numbers of false positive referrals. This problem might apply to particular sources of referrals (for example, referrals from mental health services but not referrals from primary care), therefore, ideally testing should have been carried out in representative samples of the population in which it will need to be used.

It is not unusual for tests to have been evaluated only by comparing test performance in a pre-selected high risk group (for example, patients diagnosed with the condition), with a separate control group (in which the diagnosis is rare or unlikely). In such a comparison, specificity tends to be over-optimistic and the optimal threshold recommended for the test may be too high or low. Readers requiring further guidance on how to inform referral decisions for their clinic population may find that the advice of a clinical epidemiologist will be useful in deciding whether to adopt a test routinely. The problem of test validity discussed here is very common throughout medicine, but it has not always been sufficiently well understood in the field of adult autism services.

Tests used to help inform a decision whether to seek an assessment for autism

Currently available tests relevant to deciding when an assessment is worth seeking are listed in Table 5.1. Further information on measures, used in clinical assessment, will be found in Chapters 7, 8 , and 9; information on tests that may have value in assessing outcome are set out in Chapter 11 on detailed needs assessment.

Given that the diagnosis of autism has historically rested very much on observation of psychological development, particularly in childhood, it should not be surprising that tests for possible autism have only recently begun to be developed and evaluated for use with adults. The UK National Institute for Clinical (Care) Excellence systematically reviewed the available tests (National Institute for Health and Clinical Excellence (Great Britain), 2012); updates of the NICE review are scheduled five-yearly. No test could be recommended by NICE (2012) for cost-effectiveness, for use in primary care. At that time no tests had been evaluated for use in populations, such as adults attending mental health services, which

Table 5.1 Test questionnaires to inform a decision to seek a referral for an assessment for possible autism in an adult*

Title	Development	Description, purpose, and suitability according to age group (where known)	Evaluation where known	Total number of questions and items
Australian Scale for Asperger syndrome (ASAS)	Developed by Tony Attwood (http://www.aspennj.org/pdf/information/articles/australian-scale-for-asperger-syndrome.pdf).	A parent/teacher rating tool designed for **older children** who do not have a significant degree of intellectual disability (but because of its public availability, it is used more widely). It does not give scores or a cut-off, but does alert individuals, parents, and teachers to the possibility of autism.	–	24 graded questions and a 10-item behavioural checklist.
Gilliam Autism Rating Scale (GARS and GARS-2)	GARS-2 is a revised version. To be added to.	A parental/teacher checklist for people **up to 22 years of age**. It is advocated as a well-standardized USA screening instrument.	Published research indicates that it is insufficiently sensitive to be an effective discriminant of ASD. It is not yet clear whether the concerns about the earlier instrument have been resolved.	42 items divided into three sections (stereotyped behaviours, communications, and social interactions) and takes 5–10 minutes to complete and score.

Social Communication Questionnaire (SCQ)	(Previously known as the Autism Screening Questionnaire.) Developed from the Autism Diagnostic Interview—revised (ADI-R). Developed by Michael Rutter, Anthony Bailey, and Catherine Lord (www.hogrefe.co.uk/social-communication-questionnaire-scq.html).	It comes in two versions (lifetime and current) for use with people over 4 years of age. It should be completed by the parent/carer (Berument et al, 1999).	–	40-item questionnaire.
Social Responsiveness Scale—2 (SRS—2). (previously known as the Social Reciprocity Scale.)	Developed by John M. Constantino (www4.parinc.com/products/Product.aspx?ProductID=SRS-2).	To be completed by a parent/teacher in less than 20 minutes. There is an adult module for those over 18 years of age. It gives a total score as well as scoring on five subscales (Constantino and Gruber, 2002).	–	65-item questionnaire
Autism Spectrum Quotient (AQ) and Autism Spectrum Quotient-10 (AQ-10)	Developed by comparing diagnosed clinic cases of autism with normal control groups (students, GP listed adults). The AQ (or AQ-50) and the AQ-10 are produced by the Autism Research Centre (www.autismresearchcentre.com/arc_tests).	The AQ is a self-report questionnaire that is intended to provide a summary score that indicates the likelihood of ASD. In practice, it requires a degree of insight; completion by an informant will often give a higher score (more autistic). The AQ-10 uses 10 of the AQ's more discriminatory items and is recommended by NICE (National Institute for Health and Clinical Excellence, 2012) to identify those who should have a more comprehensive assessment for autism.	Independent evaluations: it has a low specificity when used in the general population (Brugha et al, 2012). Is more accurate and cost effective in **adult** mental health service patients (Tyrer et al, 2013).	50-item full version. 20- and 10-item versions available.

(continued)

Table 5.1 Continued

Title	Development	Description, purpose, and suitability according to age group (where known)	Evaluation where known	Total number of questions and items
Ritvo Autism Asperger Diagnostic Scale—Revised (RAADS—R)	Recently developed	To be completed by the clinician, but can be self-completed by the patient with guidance. Authors do not claim that it is an alternative to a diagnostic assessment.	Developers report an acceptable level of sensitivity and specificity in **adult** patients with autism attending a mental health service when compared with normal adult controls (Ritvo et al, 2011). Independent evaluation in **adults** in contact with mental health services shows acceptable, and cost effective sensitivity and specificity with a higher than recommended cut-off of 120 or greater.	80-item structured questionnaire

Social and Communication Disorders Checklist (SCDC)	A screening questionnaire for completion by parents.	Claimed to be suitable for population surveys (Skuse et al, 2004).	An adult version has yet to be validated. 12 items
Autism Behaviour Checklist (ABC)	Was designed for the diagnosis of autism in young children. Available from PRO-ED Inc. (www.proedinc.com/customer/ProductView.aspx?ID=4219).	For completion by parents	Claimed to have good statistical underpinning for its original purpose, and people are now experimenting with its use for **older children** (Krug et al, 1980).

***None** of these tests is suitable on its own for diagnosis, including self-diagnosis; together with an overall clinical evaluation and judgement, they may assist with referral decisions.

Source: data from: Berney et al., CR136. Psychiatric services for adolescents and adults with Asperger syndrome and other autistic-spectrum disorders, Copyright 2006, Royal College of Psychiatrists may be the population of primary interest to many readers of this chapter. However, several tests were found to be useful as an adjunct to clinical decision-making in primary care, when combined with the kinds of descriptive and background information already set out in this chapter. At the time of writing there does not appear to be any change to the available evidence base.

Two tests that can be completed by the adult (self-report) are the Autism Spectrum Quotient (Baron-Cohen et al. 2001) and the Ritvo Asperger Autism Diagnostic Scale Revised (RAADS-R; Ritvo et al. 2011) (the RAADS-R can be administered by a professional or can be self-completed). Several tests are mentioned in the NICE review that should be completed by an observer, such as a parent or a carer. Since the publication of the NICE Guidance in 2012, the author's research team has completed evaluations of both tests (Tyrer et al. 2013) for use within general adult mental health patient populations. Full length versions of both tests can be recommended in this population as cost effective in determining whether there is an increased likelihood that the patient has an autism spectrum disorder, for which a specialist diagnostic assessment may be worthwhile. Both tests appear to show excellent negative predictive value; accordingly, a negative test suggests that the patient would be very unlikely to receive a diagnosis of autism if referred for an assessment. However, in the case of the RAADS-R the decision threshold recommended by the original developers was not supported; a higher threshold was required in order to maximize specificity and sensitivity (Tyrer et al. 2013). The threshold recommended by the developers of the AQ was found to be cost effective. Another recent study that included referrals from primary care suggested that the AQ did not contribute usefully to predicting an autism diagnosis in such settings (Ashwood, 2016).

Finding and choosing a suitable service to which to refer

The type and location of specialist service to which the patient is to be referred is an important consideration. The following points are based mainly on the experience of the author working in England, where services that are publically funded are being developed, but this may not apply elsewhere. In parts of the world where there is growing provision in the independent sector it may be prudent to identify an independent organization that evaluates the standards and quality of such services before choosing which to refer to. However, some points made here may be of wider general applicability.

Many areas operate services for adults with moderate to profound levels of intellectual disability (Davidson et al. 2015), and some of these services may be willing to offer an assessment to an adult who is more able and who is suspected of having an autism spectrum disorder. It is often the case that service contracts with commissioners ('payers') preclude intellectual disability services from offering post-diagnostic care, or follow-up. Furthermore, staff working with intellectually-disabled adults, may be clinically less familiar with the more able population, which could lead both to some autism symptoms being overlooked, or rated as insignificant. Similarly, they may be less aware of options for further assessment and for post-diagnostic support, so that although a diagnosis may be correct, the needs of the patient may be more difficult to meet in his or her community.

In some geographic areas assessment services do not have medical or psychology input, or otherwise lack experience in differentiating autism from other mental or behavioural disorders. Such services may have difficulty in filtering for patients seeking a diagnostic label, such as 'Asperger syndrome', who may have been diagnosed with other forms of behavioural or mental disorder that overlap with autism. Important alternative explanations for a presentation may be overlooked and false positive diagnoses on the autism spectrum may be more likely to occur, leading to further difficulties later on. Since psychiatric comorbidity is common in patients seeking an autism assessment, a good working knowledge of general mental health services and referral routes, is important. Before choosing a service it is important to seek advice and to have advance knowledge of the staffing, and the expertise of such services.

Where services do not exist locally, out-of-area referral may be the only option. Regional and national referral centres with considerable specialist experience may be the best or only option. Before deciding to make a referral, the kinds of recommendations that could follow if autism is diagnosed should be considered. Out of area (i.e. regional or national) centres will normally be able to provide general information of this kind.

Experiences and expectation of the process of referral

The expectations of patients and carers need to be carefully considered and discussed before finally deciding to make a referral. Hence, the importance of the question 'what do you hope to get out of an assessment?'

Patients (and carers) will often mention the possibility of support becoming available. It is not unusual for considerable frustration to be caused to individual patients, and their families and carers, on returning with a diagnosis to their home setting, to find that the help and services recommended are not available there. Ideally, assessment services should be linked to local provision of post-diagnostic care and support (Chapters 13–14). In some areas, such as in England, educational services may be able to offer support throughout college years for the age group 16–25 years, funded by local education authorities. Similar considerations may apply to the independent sector, which may be able to provide short- and medium-term support and remedies, but not necessarily the long-term support that an adult with significant autistic problems may require. Experience in England provides a number of examples of an imbalance between the ease with which services can be found to undertake short-term assessment, and 'habilitation', in contrast to the considerable difficulties encountered in trying to find a return care pathway to the patient's home community.

If there are known issues of risk to the person themselves or to others (usually to the family), or issues of vulnerability and self-neglect, this information may help to accelerate the timing of completion of a requested assessment. During years in employment, a referral may come through occupational health services; there is considerable potential for such services to liaise constructively between representatives of an employer and the patient, and those supporting him or her. If an individual has been assessed in childhood, or in the early teen years, a referral may come in the form of a request for assistance with the transition to early adult services. Arguably, the same issues will apply in relation to an adult nearing retirement age who is making the transition into services for older and for frail adults.

At the time of writing, although the number of specialist clinics available for offering assessments is growing rapidly throughout England, demand for such specialist clinics is exceeding their supply. Some may also increasingly be asked to see patients who do not have autism, but who often do have complex problems in communication with others and in social functioning, for example, due to ADHD, or, as mentioned above, a form of personality disorder, such as borderline personality disorder (and see Chapter 10).

Chapter 6

Initial assessment ('Triage')

Background

Initial or triage assessments are preferably led by clinicians experienced in assessing adults both with autism and adults with a range of mental disorders, because complex diagnostic considerations are involved.[1] Accepting a patient for a long and complex assessment, where it is unnecessary, is wasteful and may complicate matters unhelpfully if their difficulties are due to other reasons. This chapter may also be useful to clinicians, at earlier stages of learning about autism, as a step to follow before asking for advice from a more specialist colleague. On balance, if in doubt about whether or not your patient is on the spectrum, do consider seeking more experienced advice before taking a decision to rule out autism and informing the patient that you do not think they have it. Patients with autism who have been responded to incorrectly in this way, perhaps by an inexperienced colleague, may turn to other less appropriate sources of advice, and suffer from the delay in obtaining correct advice and support. Be prepared to be open about being unsure.

Consider what people say and do, which points to non-autistic explanations and to those that point to possible autism

Throughout an initial short or triage assessment, it is important to make observations and to use questions that can point to *and* also away from the possibility of autism. Equally, it is important to listen, note, observe responses, and behaviours from both points of view. It is very easy to slip into the position that everyone referred to such a clinic is somewhere on

---

[1] This will usually be a psychiatrist with training in neurodevelopmental psychopathology and treatment, but there are also clinical psychologists who have a similar range of training and expertise to offer, over and above standard training in their discipline.

the autism spectrum. In most parts of the world, diagnostic resources are limited and it is important that they are channelled to those who are most likely to gain, rather than be disadvantaged by a diagnosis and the action of others, to support an affected individual. Audit and professional peer group activities are an important underpinning to the role of the assessor (see Conclusions to the final chapter).

Considering alternatives to autism and the influence of comorbidities

Within a triage clinic, it is important to become vigilant about alternative, non-autistic, conditions that seem to result in a referral to autism diagnostic services. Alternatives may be neurodevelopmental or adult 'functional' psychiatric disorders. Experience in such clinic settings point to conditions such as undiagnosed ADHD, chronic depression, personality disorder, including mild to moderate sociopathy (in a few cases with ongoing contact with the criminal justice system), or unrecognized mild intellectual disability (Chapter 10, Box 10.1).

Triage clinic format

The format of an initial assessment, or triage, meeting consists of the four steps set out in Box 6.1. When written referrals are received, those that are clearly inappropriate or misdirected are dealt with in writing and not

---

Box 6.1 Four steps in an initial or triage assessment

- Initial greeting and meeting with the patient, and introductions to any accompanying person/s.
- Interview with the patient exploring reasons for seeking an assessment, including consideration of non-autism explanations for a referral.
- Interview with informant/s/carers with particular emphasis on early life. development compared with other children they have observed growing up.
- Conclusion of initial meeting; agreement on next steps to be followed; clarification of expectations; completion of paperwork or agreement on arrangements for doing so.

considered further (unless re-referred with a clearer set of reasons). Most referrals are accepted and an initial appointment is sent within 6–8 weeks, addressed to the patient.

Patients are told in writing that it is very important that they are accompanied by an adult, such as a parent or other family member, or someone who has known them a long time. The need for early developmental information has been strongly emphasized on many occasions in this book. However, some patients do attend on their own—and much of the initial short meeting may be spent explaining how important it is for the clinic doctor to also speak with someone who knows them well, preferably an older family member, and sometimes in negotiating who that could be and how to involve them acceptably. Most patients are accompanied.

Ideally, patients should also be informed in writing and requested to confirm they will attend or their appointment will be cancelled. Good administrative back-up is important so that an attempt may be made to contact those who have not responded, to check if they are coming. ADHD is common in this referral population—a strong signal for possible ADHD is missing appointments. Many clinics send a text to or phone the patient the day before an appointment.

Meeting and greeting

Experience in adult autism diagnostic clinics has taught that initial observations and impressions can be very useful. In contrast, in adult psychiatry settings, initial impressions may be quite misleading.[2] That initial meeting in a waiting room for an autism clinic can be very informative, which is illustrated with the help of some contrasting scenarios. The observations to make are as set out earlier in Chapter 2 (alerting characteristics, Box 2.1), in this chapter (Table 6.1), and in Chapter 9 (focusing in particular on non-verbal communication signs, such as gaze, gesture, vocal intonation, and facial expression).

The doctor greets and introduces themselves by name and asks, by name, if the patient is in the waiting room. There are two fairly distinct scenarios one can observe in the clinic waiting area, at this point (not all first encounters are as clear as these contrasting examples):

1. Several people in the waiting room respond and it is not clear, at first, which one is the named patient. One of the group looks directly at the doctor (with good gaze and engagement), speaks up, and clarifies who the patient is. The doctor then addresses the patient and asks, 'who have

---

[2] Masked depression being an obvious example in the mental health clinic context.

Table 6.1 Observing non-verbal communication during a short initial, triage meeting

Opportunities for observation	How or where to create the opportunity to make observations
First encounters with patient and accompanying adults	For example, in the waiting room before the assessment begins
Responses to structured focused direct questions	Asking very factual direct and largely closed questions, such as what is your date of birth
Responses to comment, informality, chat	• Ask the patient to describe a non-routine event, such as a weekend break, recent holiday, going to a public event • Pass a remark, interrupt with a comment, suddenly change the subject • At the end of the triage session observe the patient's non-verbal behaviour while in the consulting room with carers they have chosen to bring with them to the clinic

you brought with you?', while glancing at the others in the group. One of the others in the group will often then say 'I'm X's mother' (or partner, or sister, or friend, or wife).

2. One person looks directly at the doctor and clarifies 'I'm "X"'. The doctor also says 'who have you brought with you?' And X introduces those accompanying them as parent, partner, friend, etc. The accompanying person(s) do not step in or interrupt.

There are also other, less clear cut scenarios. Which of these two do you, the reader, think might be a patient on the autism spectrum and which is less likely to be? Answers can be found at the end of this chapter—have a good guess before looking. It is not as easy as it seems—initial impressions can also be highly misleading. Do not worry if you get it wrong.

It is explained that the patient will be interviewed first.[3] It is important, as it were, to put the patient to the test, seeing them alone initially. Then with her or his permission, those accompanying will be interviewed. The doctor

---

[3] At a later full assessment meeting, the informants are seen at length first. However, it can be a great advantage and is certainly only fair to the patient that they be seen initially at the first contact meeting. After all, how else would one have their consent and how else would one know what they want?

asks the patient is that acceptable? A not uncommon response is that the patient does not wish to be seen alone; they want to be accompanied by a parent or carer. Rarely, is it necessary to accept that the patient will not be seen alone, in which case the carer sits in, but is clearly requested not to respond to any questions unless the patient clearly asks the carer to do so. Carers are often surprised by how well patients manage a first meeting with a complete stranger.

Those of one's colleagues who have a good deal of experience in running such clinics will also talk about the importance and value of first impressions—particularly where it soon turns out that the patient is, clearly, quite significantly affected by autism. Looking across a waiting room (such waiting rooms are often being used by other services and clinics at the same time), it is often possible to spot a patient who one immediately thinks, (s)he is very possibly on the spectrum, (although that does not necessarily mean that (s)he is coming to the autism diagnostic clinic).

Normally, in a first meeting with a patient who may never have come to see a psychiatrist previously, the rule is to make the encounter as free of anxiety as possible for the patient. That is the case here, of course. By the end of an initial autism triage assessment, the patient will have been seen alone and will have been seen with their carers present, with the doctor. Being seen with carers, who are others they have handpicked to represent them, should provide an opportunity to evaluate how they respond to more relaxed 'chit chat' and informal remarks (coming from the doctor), and to check how they use eye gaze to interact with more than one other person in the consultation room. In general, within an autism assessment, we want to observe patients both 'at their best' and also in a state in which they are 'put on the spot', i.e. are perhaps more anxious.[4] The examiner needs to quite deliberately create these contrasting scenarios, formal and informal, which may differ from the usual consultation style. In principle, signs of autism ought to be present across multiple contexts—if signs are no longer present in a more relaxed context, which opens up the possibility that there may be reasons other than autism for that person being advised to seek an assessment.

---

[4] It may be that it requires anxiety to over-ride someone's learned interview skills to reveal their autism. Conversely, carers sometimes comment that it is only when their offspring or partner is relaxed that repetitive behaviours and stereotypies are observed.

Questions to be asked of a patient at a first short meeting

Box 6.2 sets out some of the issues to be considered in what is, necessarily, a short meeting with the patient, almost always alone.

Any of the example questions that follow may generate symptoms suggestive of autism or of other conditions. In this section, the assessment process will be focused on more, and the value of each question will be noted in determining whether a more detailed assessment might need to be arranged. In the chapters that follow we will focus more on those symptoms and how to weigh up their significance.

Having explained that we are having a short meeting to help us decide what we might need to do next, a good beginning could be to ask the following question.

Do you know why it has been suggested that you should come to this clinic?

This may seem an odd question (an accompanying trainee may sometimes seem a bit taken aback by this). This question can be put in several other ways.

Do you know why you are here? Did your doctor say why they thought it might help to come here? Do you know what this clinic is for?

Box 6.2 Issues to be considered during a first meeting with the patient

- Benefits and risks for the patient.
- Their own views about their difficulties.
- Whether (s)he is able to fit into the social world around themselves.
- Whether a detailed assessment is necessary and at this time.
- Consideration of alternative reasons for a referral, including a mental or behavioural disorder.
- The involvement of carers and informants, and consent to retain third party information.
- Clinician observations of patient interaction behaviour and use of non-verbal skills (see also Table 6.1).

Which of these questions to choose will depend, in part, on the information in the referral and any reference there to the patient's role in the request.

For the autistic person it is a form of questioning that appeals to their strengths as reasoning and as logically directed persons—who only do things because it makes sense to do so.

This line of questioning may also tease out the person presenting to the clinic who is very keen to have the 'Asperger' or 'autism' label, who has already been given other diagnostic labels that they find less acceptable. The following could also be the first question to ask.

What do you hope to get out of an assessment?

This is a very important question.

The obvious answer often conveys a wish for certainty. A patient might express it thus (at this stage, it is not known if this person will receive an autism diagnosis): 'if I have it I have an explanation, something to say to others'. 'If I don't then I'm left as I am, seen by others as a difficult person'.

Patients will often say that with a diagnosis there will surely be some form of help. It is also a question one often returns to, towards the end of a detailed assessment that might take place and be concluded a long time after the first contact.

What sorts of problems have you had, not just recently, but also going back into childhood?

This kind of question is often used to rescue the initial meeting from getting stuck with little or no information emerging, of descriptive or of explanatory value. It is, of course, open-ended, which is desirable. Again, it is therefore an opportunity to help differentiate those needing further scrutiny from those who may not need it.

Have you read about autism (or Asperger syndrome) or seen the subject in television documentaries, or in newspaper or magazine articles?

What was your reaction? Did they describe anything that reminded you of yourself as a person?

These can be very revelatory questions. They are particularly useful in interviewing parents and carers.

Has this affected you when at school, college, or work?

Questions can also be asked about routines, and repetitive and rigid behaviours (both of the patient and of carers).

Friends, marriage, social interaction difficulties

It is of central importance to ask about social contact the person has with friends. Probing and following up what they say is vital. The reply 'I have lots of friends' tells you nothing and may lead the examiner astray. In autism, contact with friends tends to be very infrequent, even when there is no practical reason why it might be difficult to keep in touch. Check the meaning of contact. It may be mainly online. If online, explore what contacts are for—they may be just for the purposes of electronic gaming or a narrow interest. They may involve a richness of sharing of life—as one would expect in the non-autistic relationship.

Other issues

At any time in this first, short meeting, follow-up questions may be asked on possible treatment history, relevant comorbid explanations, such as obsessive compulsive disorder, ADHD, emotional disorders, psychosis, behavioral problems, etc. (see Chapter 10).

Positive responses to self-completed test questions are particularly useful if they seem to point to ADHD. The ASRS (Kessler et al. 2005) shows promise at picking out patients who, on questioning, are found to have significant ADHD symptoms.[5]

Many patients coming to the clinic have been taking antidepressant medication and some anxiolytics. Often the former have not helped; sometimes the latter have helped and have become difficult to manage without. A few may have been inpatients (requests for past records are an important part of each stage of any assessment process).

Observations on social communication

During the meeting with the patient, it is important to consciously return to an observational mode and to make notes. Table 6.1 summarizes opportunities to observe non-verbal communication and Table 6.2 lists the different modes of non-verbal communication to focus on.

In Chapter 9, we will also explore how both autism, and other mental and neurological disorders can give rise to variations in non-verbal expression and communication. Importantly, we will also discuss gender differences. At the time of writing, there is a growing consensus, not yet systematically tested in research, that women, seemingly, are better at learning to recognize and manage their non-verbal signs effectively, more so than men of the

---

[5] However, without a formal test evaluation in this setting one cannot predict if true cases have been missed due to low test sensitivity.

Table 6.2 Modes of non-verbal communication to note in observing a patient at a first contact

Mode	Points to observe
Gaze	Difficulties in establishing and maintaining eye gaze
Gesture	Lack of gesture
Facial expression	Lack of expressiveness
Vocal intonation	Too loud or too quiet, monotony

same ability level. They may, therefore, effectively conceal such difficulties from observers. Research, discussed in Chapter 3, suggests that this ability is absent in intellectually disabled women, in whom the prevalence of autism is just as high as in intellectually disabled men (Brugha et al. 2016). Failure to consider this could lead to some women being denied more detailed assessment.

Issues of consent

All patients are asked to consider whether they are willing to involve others in the assessment process. Consent in writing is sought, obtained, recorded, and filed. This should include a careful check of the patient's understanding of the meaning and possible eventual outcomes of deciding to involve others. This population is more likely to include individuals with some degree of learning difficulty; hence, the importance of checking that consent is valid, understood, and freely given. Written information should also be provided for the patient to take away that explains reasons for involving informants, as well as reasons for other procedures followed by the clinic.

Reasons for meeting informants and parents

One might ask why it is so important to invite parents or alternative informants? Early and formative learning experiences may provide a valuable illustrative lesson. A patient later diagnosed with autism, seen for about a year and failing to engage much, if at all, in communication, proved to be a challenging puzzle. The patient's mother was very insistent that her son continue to be seen. She was then interviewed by Dr Lorna Wing in her capacity as a trainer in autism of training grade clinicians. Dr Wing then spoke to the patient. The impression conveyed was like turning the lights on in a dark unlit room. It was plainly obvious that this man had been totally

> **Box 6.3 Issues to be considered in a first meeting with carers and informants**
>
> - Principle concerns of carers. For example, concerns about the patient's capacity for independence, and any associated vulnerabilities and consequent risk issues.
> - Short account of early development of the patient from childhood onwards.
> - If the informant is a contemporary of the patient (sibling, partner, spouse) an account of the patient when functioning at his or her 'best' ever compared with now.
> - If necessary, advice of contemporary informants on who else might also be able to provide information on early childhood development.

different socially from his childhood peers, but academically capable. Dr Wing spoke loudly and directly to the young man, and he responded equally clearly, without any of the hesitation or apparent temerity that had marked his previous clinic contacts. For the first time, communication had been established clearly with and by a doctor who knew how to compensate for his impaired communication.

Experience shows that 20 minutes spent with a parent is worth two hour-long meetings with a patient on the autism spectrum.[6] Parents of disabled offspring have a depth of knowledge and wisdom about their adult child that we can never hope to achieve. It is vital to respect that and not to dismiss it.[7] The issues to be considered in the meeting with informants are set out in Box 6.3.

However, talking to parents may not always be helpful. A difficulty can arise in that parents can idealize their children and are reluctant to say anything negative when the offspring is clearly quite disabled. This is not always obvious. A 'give away' is the parent who repeatedly remonstrates that 'my son is not abnormal'—'there is nothing wrong with him, Doctor'. Informants who are close relatives may well be on the spectrum themselves—they can be misleading if it means that they see little unusual in their offspring. More

---

[6] However, see Chapter 8 on newly emerging and potentially effective patient interview techniques.

[7] Such parents often report accounts of their child's difficulties being dismissed by professionals.

psychologically minded parents may also divert the discussion (and it may come across as a discussion) into various less directly relevant areas of possible early psychological development. It may be difficult to pin them down to a few key questions of direct relevance to possible autism.

Questions for informants such as parents and non-parental carers[8]

After an interview with the patient of about 15–20 minutes, the informant(s) is or are seen. It is important to start by explaining to informants that the meeting will be short and that only a few key points can be considered. Carers and other informants may also have issues and concerns (Box 6.3). If a subsequent more detailed assessment (Chapter 7) is needed, there will be more time available then.

In an initial consultation there are quite a lot of points to try to cover quickly with parents and/or other informants, where available and where feasible. Not all can be covered in such a short meeting. Most of these will need to be refreshed and expanded upon in a more detailed assessment meeting at a later time, if it is decided that one is needed (Chapters 7–9).

What are your main concerns now?

Parents are often concerned about whether their offspring will be able to manage without them in the future.[9] Such concerns by parents must be respected. This question can also be useful in pointing to relatively few concerns. It can light up that the concerns only began in recent years for which there may be two contrasting explanations. First, this may point to a late onset mental disorder and possibly a personality change, rather than to a developmental disorder such as autism. Second, it could point to the alternative of a late acknowledgement of the need for an assessment, as parents realize how impermanent their situation is when their lives are interrupted by retirement, marital problems, or changes in funding for a placement.

This first question to carers about concerns may also alert to the possibility of risk, as in vulnerability and, as in risk to others, usually in the family. Information on problems in behaviour in childhood and now, in public and in the home, should also be enquired about when undertaking a more detailed assessment (see Chapter 7).

---

[8] Siblings, spouses, and friends can be a helpful alternative to unavailable parental informants.

[9] If the only surviving parent is ill and facing a short life-span, the referral and assessment, if possible, should be expedited sooner.

Some of the questions listed earlier for the interview with the patient, appropriately reworded, are valuable in bringing out descriptions that could point to autism. Equally, they may point to alternative explanations, such as a later developing depressive disorder, or later developing personality and adjustment difficulties.

Earliest concerns

Ask when concerns first arose. Ask if help was sought. Often this can lead to mention of problems with speech, and the provision of Speech and Language Therapy (SALT), around the time of starting at school, at 4 or 5 years of age. Ask was there ever a time when there were no concerns?

Examples of early behaviour with peers (strangers)

It is often revealing to take the parent/s back to when they first brought their child to a nursery, pre-school, or crèche, to ask them how easily the child fitted in with his/her own age group. Another potentially revealing line is to ask what happened on holidays—did the child prefer to stay with parents and carers, to join in with and play with one or more other children of approximately their own age, or to play alone regardless of whether other children were there? The latter is more likely in a child who has problems on the autism spectrum. A child that makes the effort to find others to play with is very unlikely to have social difficulties now because of purely developmental reasons.

Reaction to first reading about autism: 'might this be my child?'

This question is useful early in an interview with parents or with another adult companion or carer (as it can be when talking to the patient). The reaction the parent experienced can be quite a strong one, in a case of autism. 'That's him'. 'Suddenly it all made sense'. Alternatively, the response may be that some elements applied and some did not. One would follow-up asking for examples and not prompting, if possible.

Impact of symptoms on the person's life

Impact on life and on current functioning is particularly important. It may be substantial or it can be very slight. Sometimes we see people who are functioning well. For them having a diagnosis is mainly a matter of personal curiosity; it is not strictly a health issue. In a busy and, sometimes inadequately funded public clinic, we may have to be firm about the amount of time we can give to such perfectly legitimate questions. Sometimes in those instances, a suggestion may be put that there are other settings and other professionals[10] they might chose to turn to in order to take that forward.

In contrast, adults on the spectrum with significant problems will describe breakdown in school attendance (or periods of employment in adulthood that are not sustained). Parents may describe being left with no choice but to home school their child, dropping out of college or university, as they could not cope, due to the many symptoms of the condition. Issues of risk, including vulnerability, may also be mentioned.

The following questions may provide some initial pointers (the wording is addressed to the caregiver; it can be reworded for the interview with the patient).

Does (s)he live with family, with others, or alone? How well does (s)he manage?

Does (s)he have to rely on other people or can you manage alone?

These questions are to help determine how much the person has developed or may be capable of developing independence. In the assessment clinic population, people on the spectrum who are still living in the parental home, often have the range of skills required to function independently, but may not use them except when asked or prompted to by a carer. These questions may reveal if the person has insight or fails to due to considering it unimportant, problems with planning, or lack of interest or energy.

Information showing significant impact of symptoms on functioning is required for the diagnosis of autism spectrum disorder under DSM-5.[11] This makes sense as there are quite possibly many adults with some symptoms of autism who are functioning satisfactorily throughout most of their adult lives for whom the diagnostic label of autism may be of questionable value.

Informants who are partners or peers of the referred patient

It is not unusual for referrals to be in relation to an adult in a long-term relationship or marriage. This suggests a higher level of functioning than one might think possible with an autism diagnosis. They are usually accompanied by the spouse or partner (parents may need to be brought into the

---

[10] Such a client might be pointed to an appropriate professional body for information on sources of guidance, such as, in the UK, the British Psychological Society.

[11] The APA DSM-5 autism spectrum advisory sub-panel had to argue strongly for this stipulation.

> **Box 6.4 Range of outcomes of an initial brief (triage) assessment**
>
> - Definite autism (subject to completing checks on early development) and only to be decided in clear-cut cases by an experienced autism clinician.
> - Definitely not autism (requiring advice on where to go next, including a different line of assessment).
> - Requires a detailed assessment (explanation of what is involved and length of delay to completion).

process). The partner may describe great difficulties in the relationship, but know little of the person's childhood. Difficulties in such adult relationships are also common in the context of other forms of mental disorder, notably personality disorder, affective disorder, or alcohol and drug misuse.

In a short triage meeting there will not be time to explore such complex issues; again, it is important to avoid giving the impression that such a discussion is possible within a short initial meeting.[12]

Be prepared to take an open-minded view of the reasons for a referral (as in this potentially more involved kind of example). A referral can omit information pointing to possible alternative explanations for social functioning difficulties. If possible, as in a referral from a colleague in the same organization, try to see the original case records completed by the referrer, as these may not be sent with the request to see the patient.

Concluding the meeting with informants and patient present together

The patient is then invited back to join the meeting with carers and the meeting is concluded with agreement and clarification on next steps (Box 6.4). These can range from immediate discharge, through discussion of the possible need for a later more detailed assessment. An immediate confirmation of a diagnosis on the autism spectrum, in cases that are obvious and straightforward is less common (subject to final confirmation when details

---

[12] This is yet another reason why such clinical work is better undertaken by an experienced practitioner. Inexperience could lead to a challenging scenario not relevant to the meeting's purpose.

of early development are described in documentation to be completed by informants such as parents). Procedures to be followed in the case of a diagnosis are set out in Part III of this book.

A final opportunity to evaluate the patient may be the clinician's observations of how the patient and informants behave as they leave. Patients with autism often do not use gaze or engage by looking back at the doctor, as they turn to leave the consulting room. Nor do they shake hands. Informants often notice, as they look to the clinician one more time, as they are leaving. Hand-shaking comes naturally to most carers, as if automatically—in contrast to the hand-shake of the autistic patient that is often quite hesitant, 'forced', and artificial feeling.

In conclusion, deciding on whether a full assessment is needed

Box 6.4 sets out the three most likely outcomes of an initial assessment (a fourth may be to discuss this with a colleague before deciding which to follow).

A decision to diagnose autism on the basis of a short meeting, albeit with good referral information and well-documented past records, should only be made by an experienced clinician, and then only in cases that are clear and obvious. It is very important that the need, if any, for a detailed assessment is considered before arriving at a conclusion based on a short evaluation.

What are the benefits and risks for the patient, and what is their view? If you are confident that the patient has autism, postponing making the diagnosis 'official', while awaiting a detailed assessment (in some services there may be a delay of a year or longer before this can be completed), will delay beginning to make acceptance and support possible for the patient. On the other hand, a diagnosis by a psychiatrist has an incredible 'stickiness' property about it. It can be very hard to reverse an incorrect diagnosis at a later time. Clinical diagnostic services should provide for the possibility of offering a second independent opinion.

Being able to diagnose an obvious case of autism at that first contact, assuming it is correct, has potential advantages. It means the person can begin to get help without further delay. In Part III we will set out what that help and support can mean.

In at least half of all referrals, it is not easy to tell a great deal in a 20–25-minute meeting with patient and any carers, particularly if the patient is not 'low functioning'. In such cases, it is right to engage in a much more detailed assessment process, as set out in the remainder of Part II, before making a definitive decision. Often comorbidities complicate the picture and require a meticulous teasing apart of the evidence.

If more detailed assessment is anticipated, prepare the patient and carers to expect what will follow and when. Be concrete and allow time to go into detail. Who will need to be involved? When will it happen? When will an appointment be sent? What else does the patient need to do (i.e. complete test questionnaires)? What else do the carers, and particularly parents or older relatives, need to do (complete test questionnaires covering early development and functioning)?

In those cases where autism is obviously absent, there is still some work to do. What was the basis for the decision to seek an assessment? What might be seen by the patient, their doctor, their carer, or by others, as to the value of a diagnosis? What are the motivations of patients and carers? What alternative ways might there be of directly addressing the patient's problems? An obvious difficulty here is that you don't have time in a short appointment to look into all the alternatives. This is why it is important, when offering triage meetings, that you make it clear at the start that, 'If we don't think you need our service further, we will try to point you in a different direction, in the hope of finding what you need'.

Sometimes we are faced with a more acute situation where the person is in crisis, may be in trouble with the law, facing the breakdown of a care structure or care relationship, a falling-apart marriage, or other long-term supportive relationship. Whatever the decision, and it may be that they need a more detailed assessment, it is important to be flexible about making the necessary arrangements more quickly, and keeping other professional colleagues aware of that, including the referring doctor. There should be a careful check that physical health has been monitored and identified needs followed up.

Learning about autism for the first time, as an experienced general psychiatrist, should include opportunities to see and take part in conducting detailed assessment procedures under supervision, even if one is not to become a specialist in this area. In particular, this should cover the classic and probably the most reliable route to a diagnostic assessment of autism, by means of a developmental history, which is described in the next chapter.

But before moving on—have you checked your results on that waiting room quiz?

View the results now.

Appendix to Chapter 6. Result of 'waiting room quiz'

Table 6.3 Waiting room scenario. Answer to the question at the beginning of Chapter 6, which one might be on the autism spectrum and which not?

Scenario	More likely explanation for scenario
1. Several people respond and at first it is not clear which one is the named patient. One of the group clarifies who it is. The doctor addresses him or her and asks, 'who have you brought with you?', while looking about at the others in the group. One of the others in the group will often then say 'I'm X's mother' (or partner, or sister, or friend).	The patient in this case has little or no sense of how to behave in this unusual context. (S)he is accustomed to carers taking all responsibility for dealing with authority figures and 'sits back' waiting for a prompt. Carers know to step in on behalf of the patient, in this case, by beginning to make introductions. The patient in this case is more likely to be on the autism spectrum.
2. One person looks directly at the doctor and clarifies 'I'm "X"'. The doctor also says 'who have you brought with you?' X introduces those accompanying them as parent, partner, friend, etc.	The person responding to the doctor's initial greeting is most likely neurotypical, understands the context, and instinctively reacts appropriately.
Other. Various other less obvious scenarios do, of course, happen.	Not all initial encounters are easy to base a strong first impression on.

Chapter 7

Full assessment: the developmental history

Introduction

In Chapter 3 we described some of the differences in childhood and early development that are generally regarded as characteristic of the autism phenotype. Child specialists have available to them various direct observation techniques for evaluating these in a child undergoing a developmental assessment, using settings in which the child can be observed with a parent or with a peer group, engaging in play and in communication. Such early information is invaluable in determining the presence of autistic traits or of autism in adults. Here, we will explore the kinds of questions used in talking to a key informant, such as to the younger adult's parent, in determining whether early development is suggestive of autism. Box 3.2 in Chapter 3 listed the differences in development that are our 'phenotypic' signals to autism. Here, we will set out how to assess them and judge which are present to a sufficiently significant degree. In Table 5.1, we listed test questionnaires to help inform a decision to seek a referral for an assessment for possible autism in an adult. In Chapter 9 we will discuss observable signs suggestive of autism that also reflect differences in development, albeit within the short time framework of a direct clinical assessment

Methods for assessing development through the eyes of a caregiver

The developmental assessment approaches currently in use and suitable for assessing an adult, are listed in Table 7.1. Although the list includes six, the first three are later developments of one approach originated under the leadership of Lorna Wing in the 1970s. The Past and Present Behaviour Schedule[57] (PPBS[57]), containing a subset of the items covered in the DISCO, can be self-completed by informants, and then used as the basis for a semi-structured interview by the clinician. The fourth method in Table 7.1,

Table 7.1 Standardized procedures for assessing retrospectively differences in child development, as seen in adults with autism spectrum disorder

Method	Acronym	Developers
The Medical Research Council Handicaps and Behaviour Schedule, semi-structured interview*	MRC HBS	Wing and Gould
Diagnostic Interview for Social and Communication Disorders, semi-structured interview	DISCO	Wing, Gould, Leekam
The Past and Present Behaviour Schedule, self-completion questionnaire	PPBS†	Lorna Wing
Autism Diagnostic interview, revised (semi-structured interview)	ADI-R	Le Couteur, Rutter, Lord and others
Adult Asperger Assessment (combines self-completion structured questionnaires and a clinical interview with informants)	AAA	Simon Baron-Cohen
Developmental, Dimensional and Diagnostic Interview (3di) (mixed structured and semi-structured interview format developed for assessments of children—an adult adaptation is in development)	3di	David Skuse

See text for references and for explanations of differences between methods.
*The MRC-HBS is no longer in use, but a publication on it is cited in the text, for those interested.
†Copies of the PPBS can be obtained from The Lorna Wing Centre, Elliot House, 113 Mason's Hill, Bromley, Kent, BR2 9HT, UK (email: lornawingcentre@nas.org.uk).

follows broadly similar lines, but was tailored to maximize reliability and has been the most widely used in research. All are used to collect information on development in early childhood and at the age the assessment is conducted (in our case in adulthood), with the exception of the Developmental, Dimensional and Diagnostic Interview (3di) for which an adult version is in development.

The approach used in this chapter (the first three in Table 7.1) was originally developed by the late Dr Lorna Wing, with clinical psychologist Dr Judith Gould, and implemented formally in a research instrument, The Handicaps and Behaviour Schedule (Wing and Gould, 1978), under the auspices of the UK Medical Research Council (MRC-HBS). The subheadings used in this chapter (and in a slightly different arrangement in Chapter 3) are a subset of the full MRC-HBS (and its successor, referred to below, the DISCO), with the title, already mentioned above, of the Past and Present Behaviour Schedule (PPBS[57]) (Table 7.1). The PPBS was shared with the author and with other colleagues in the form of a self-report questionnaire. The purpose was to encourage parents to begin to describe the development of their child (whether the child had reached adulthood was not considered essential) as a prelude to a clinical evaluation with a psychologist or psychiatrist. It was also developed to enable parents to contribute such information if unable to attend an assessment clinic.

After Lorna retired from the MRC, her work with Judith Gould, joined by Sue Leekam and others, led to the completion of the current full implementation of this approach, the Diagnostic Interview for Social and Communication Disorders (DISCO; Wing 1993, 2000; Leekam et al. 2002; Wing et al. 2002). The DISCO not only covers developmental abnormalities in autism, in exceptionally great detail, but also covers other neurodevelopmental disorders such as, for example, attention deficit hyperactivity disorder (ADHD), tick disorder, and specific language delay. Therefore, the DISCO can be regarded as a complete neurodevelopmental disorder diagnostic instrument, in the sense that it is designed to differentiate from a range of developmental disorders that, if any, may be present in a given individual. The DISCO can be compared with a briefer, widely used research measure of development in autism, the Autism Developmental Interview (ADI; Le Couteur et al. 1989), also developed under the auspices of the UK MRC, under Michael Rutter's leadership, and currently available in its revised form (ADI-R; Lord et al. 1994), which covers only autism. The ADI-R was designed to achieve high reliability in the context of research studies, in which it has been widely used. All but two items listed in the ADI-R are covered by the more detailed DISCO, which has been taken into consideration in research-validating methods used in adult epidemiology research (Brugha et al. 2012). Of these developmental assessment approaches, the ADI-R has been by far the most widely used in research; training only takes one day. The DISCO course is spread over 4 days (split into two separate 2-day courses with a period of practice using the instrument preceding the second). The DISCO course provides an excellent overall introduction to the topic of autism, making it suitable for trainees with less knowledge of autism. Detailed technical manuals and standardized training are available, and should be completed in both methods.

The Adult Asperger Assessment (AAA) (Baron-Cohen et al. 2005) begins with the patient completing two self-report questionnaires. This is followed by an assessment interview involving a caregiver who has known the patient in childhood checking each item in the questionnaires. This highly structured approach is used by a number of other diagnostic clinics in the UK.

As use of adult assessments of the 3di (Skuse et al. 2004) is still in development, it is not possible to comment on it, although in principle, as most of the same early developmental issues are covered, it is expected to be equally useful.

Scaling-up of developmental assessments in clinical settings

In the author's clinical work, the PPBS is the method relied on the most because of its flexibility and succinctness, and because of its provenance. It should be mentioned that the DISCO is not only very thorough, but it can take many hours to complete in full. Many trained in the DISCO do not use the full version regularly, except in complex cases, where there are major issues with regard to diagnosis and, of course, in research, as in my own epidemiological studies on instrument evaluation.

In most cases, the parent or other caregiver informant will already have completed the PPBS before the full assessment takes place at the clinic.[1] Informants are then interviewed, following the structure and layout of the PPBS, as outlined here.

In this chapter, we consider pointers in assessing both childhood development and current level of functioning (a contemporary who has known the patient only as an adult can contribute to the assessment of the latter, which can be extremely useful in any assessment). Each heading and its component items is scored in terms of severity—either a minor problem or a major problem with effects on general functioning, in different contexts. Central to the evaluation is whether the problem in development was present in early life, now, at both times, or never present.

The reader should, where necessary, also refer back to the account of these developmental items in Chapter 3, for a description of the way in which development may be altered in autism. A copy of either the DISCO or the PPBS should be used in the assessment itself; it may be useful to have the PPBS[57] to hand, as the reader works through the following section of this chapter, although with Box 3.2 in Chapter 3 to refer to, it should be clear in what follows how such an assessment proceeds.

The most salient (common and useful) items will also be mentioned under each heading. Certain responses to particular items may prompt the need to

---

[1] As it is a self-completion questionnaire it is also useful in obtaining information from parents and care givers who are unable to attend the clinic with the patient.

probe and ask additional questions, which will be suggested. Advice will be given on how to assess items caregivers find particularly difficult to recall or describe. Certain questions, such as those on sensory differences, may be easier for the patient to describe. The points made are those found to be of value when talking a trainee through the developmental history in the clinic.

The work of Lorna Wing and Judith Gould is acknowledged in the original development of this approach. What follows is extensively adapted by the author of this book from their original work.

Behaviour from birth to 12 months

Parents often have difficulty in remembering phases of development in the first 12 months of life, such as whether the child held out its arms to show it was ready to be picked up (see Fig. 7.1), or showed a desire to share an object of value or interest with a carer. Although reminded of the fact, they may actually refer to seeing such behaviour later in childhood. However,

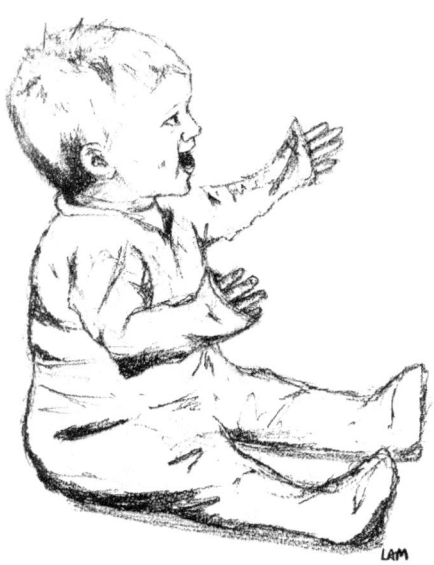

Fig. 7.1 Drawing depicting a baby aged about 10 months holding out its arms to show its carer it is ready to be picked up.
Reproduced with permission from Lucy Morton.

they do remember whether a child was demanding and constantly trying to communicate with the caregiver through gesture and gaze, or was actually more interested in objects in its surroundings and difficult to distract from such preoccupations.

Motor co-ordination and large movements

Questions about gross motor development (Chapter 3, Box 3.4) are dealt with quite straightforwardly by most caregivers. A question that uses the word 'clumsy', in relation to possible dyspraxia, might need to be explained to a parent whose first language is not English.

Fine movements and visuospatial skills

Questions about fine motor development are also dealt with quite straightforwardly by most caregivers. Poor handwriting is almost ubiquitous in this population—for recent generations of children it may be useful to add a question asking 'Did the child have access to a key board or laptop computer at school?'

Self-care skills

Most discussion on self-care skills tends to focus not so much on when the skill was acquired, but rather on whether the offspring now needs to be prompted and reminded to carry out, for example, washing and 'grooming'. Two further questions about motivation in self-care may be added to the PPBS here. 'How long are you comfortable with leaving your son/daughter alone at your home without checking in on them? For example, are you ok about taking a weekend break or a holiday, and leaving them alone at home?' 'Do you have to check him before he leaves the house in case his manner of dressing might draw unwelcome attention to him?' If the patient's manner of dressing, on the day you see them at the clinic, seems odd or unusual, ask, 'does (s)he vary what (s)he wears for example depending on the reason for going out or depending on weather and season of the year?' A reply in the negative may provide information to be coded below under 'Routines and resistance to change' (repetitive rigid behaviour). This was an issue raised in Chapter 2, Case Study C.

School work

In general, caregivers can report the child's age when it achieved certain academic standards. Unusual delay signals and a history of possible learning difficulties, should prompt further questions about whether this was recognized and, if so, what extra help was given to the child. There is often an opportunity here to identify an exceptional skill, and how it was developed or encouraged, and how it might have potential future application in employment.

Independence

Sometimes parents struggle a little to remember when their child was able or willing to go out alone, for example, to local shops. Difficulty in learning how to tell what time it is should prompt questions about the offspring's concept of time, how rigid it is, or indeed whether (s)he or he has great difficulty in using it unless everything is very precisely written down and consistently followed by everyone (s)he has to deal with.

Language and communication in childhood

In the non-intellectually disabled adult population it is unusual to come across problems with understanding of others, but problems with attention and concentration may come up and could be a signal to consider ADHD. If there is a form of repetitive speech it is important to clarify if this is echoing or topic repetition (which is far commoner).

Language and communication in adulthood: current development—questions on which an informant who has only known the patient as an adult should be able to provide observations

Up to this point, a parent or older family member, and caregiver will be required to provide information on development. The questions that follow can, however, be taken up in respect of 'current adult functioning' by a partner, sibling, or adult companion or carer, without information on childhood. When assessing older adults this may be the chronological point at which a developmental assessment begins.

Literal understanding is one of the most, if not the most, important communication item to assess in this more able, adult population, as by early adulthood it should have abated considerably, except in situations where the person, for whatever reason, is not paying attention or motivated to do so. Parents often struggle to understand what is being asked here, at first. (This may be an indication that one of two parents present at an assessment also displays autistic traits). The probe question that seems to work well here, is to ask the parent or caregiver, 'Do you need to think carefully what to say before you say it, to avoid misunderstanding?' Of course, what they say in reply might reflect very different issues, such as over sensitivity to topics that trigger anxiety or irritation (something to pick up under assessment of comorbidities, Chapter 10).

Ability to appreciate humour, or to participate and share humour, is also important and often misunderstood (often it is taken incorrectly to mean a question about whether the offspring makes jokes—individuals on the autism spectrum do make what they themselves think are funny remarks, but hardly anyone else finds them amusing). Caregivers may also be unsure, but some will point out correctly that their son or daughter laughs when everyone else does and, so, 'it's hard to tell if they get the joke'. 'Slapstick comedy' appeals to a wide range of ability levels. Humour is very cultural; this item may be one it is not possible to assess validly.

Tone of voice may need some additional explanation. Often caregivers simply do not notice how monotonous their offspring's tone of voice is, although this will be immediately obvious to peers and sometimes a trigger to bullying remarks. A voice that is too *quiet* or *loud*, however, will be obvious to caregivers. This may well be a trigger to action and possibly to a referral, if available, for speech and language therapy assessment.

The ability to hold a two-way conversation is also a crucial item to cover in any assessment (and, like tone of voice, can be assessed through direct observation). The patient may be described as responding to direct questions put to him or her, but lapsing into silence when others only make comments. It can also be difficult to assess, again all the more so, if a caregiver has the same difficulty in their own communication. An approach with the family that may be helpful is to ask them to describe whether and how their offspring fits into the general chat and conversation, when familiar relations and family friends are with them, for example, for a family gathering, birthday party, or festive occasion. One of the signs of a more subtle problem is when the person comes in 'from left of field'—cutting across the conversation because they are not good at judging how or when to join the flow. 'Does (s)he join in? Is (s)he Ok when people suddenly change topics? Does (s)he tend to try to dominate and take control when one of their particular interests is being talked about and show resistance to moving on? Can (s)he tell when others are getting bored and losing interest?'

If siblings are assisting with the assessment and, therefore, have had opportunities to observe him or her in a peer group setting outside the family home (school, parties, anywhere in the local community), ask what they have noticed. Siblings may also be acutely aware of how peers respond, an augur for ongoing difficulties in future relationships.

Body language (non-verbal communication)

Surprisingly, parents sometimes have difficulty in replying to questions about *gesture* and *variation in facial expression*. Again, this may be more so if they are still living together and simply do not notice (it is extraordinary how unaware many adults seem to be of the pervasiveness, and influence of gesture and facial expression in communication).

Often caregivers, including siblings, begin to notice non-verbal communication, more when observing their offspring interacting with their peers and other adults, when starting to live independently, but still relying on the parent for support. (What they say may not accord with what you observe—if so, consider why this may be).

We will focus on non-verbal communication in greater detail in Chapter 10.

Social interaction in childhood and now

As mentioned in Chapter 3, this aspect of development is at the heart of what we currently think about autism. Crucially, older caregivers, such as parents, have an essential role to play here in describing *early development* and providing information essential to meeting published diagnostic criteria for autism. Social interaction can also be strongly affected by any major mental disorder *in adulthood* (Chapter 10). It takes time and experience to differentiate the particular qualities of social interaction impairments in autism from those occurring in mental disorder. Several aspects can also be difficult to evaluate through caregivers, but most aspects are quite straightforward.

Social awareness, the ability to pick up on, understand, and respond appropriately to other people's feelings, is at the core of 'the social instinct' and particularly difficult for individuals on the autism spectrum to master. Parents can usually describe it, but it may be necessary sometimes to probe about what level of expression of emotion it takes to elicit a reaction, in themselves or in another family member. Parents will also describe the later development of somewhat awkward, although well intended, efforts to do so, emerging in the later teen years. Case Study D in Chapter 2 provided a possible example of a person unable to recognize the effect his behaviour has on others, although in that case there were also some signs of possibly having learning difficulties—possibly mild intellectual impairment, which also needs consideration.

Lack of interest in peers should be enquired about from early childhood. Lack of interest in interacting with other people is clearly described in depression in adulthood, and accounts based only on observation of adulthood are potentially misleading. A tendency to interact with someone much older or younger may persist, and this is something an adult observer can note without having known the patient as a child.

Social passivity, one-sided approaches or a poor understanding of how to behave in public are usually clearly described by all informants. These aspects of social interaction tend to improve with increasing maturity in a person with autism.

Parents may have limited access to information about *friendship formation* and maturity in adulthood, but will be able to give detailed accounts of difficulties up to the mid-teen years. The interview with the patient (Chapter 8) will be more useful here, provided it is sufficiently probing as mentioned already in Chapter 3. Parents normally do seem to know about bullying, although this information may have come through siblings or other informants such as teachers. A history of bullying is not a particularly useful or salient signal of autism (although it may have more value in considering autism in women).

Eye contact

As with other aspects of non-verbal communication ('Body language (non-verbal communication)'), some caregivers begin to notice problems with eye gaze, more so when observing their offspring interacting with other adults, for example, when starting to live independently. Direct observation tends to be more reliable in the adult (Chapter 9), particularly when it includes observing eye gaze when there are additional persons present.

Imagination, creativity, make believe, and pretence

Assessing imagination and pretence retrospectively can be very difficult. In an ideal world all parents would be able to show us video excerpts of their child's play.

Only parental caregivers (or sometimes grandparents) can provide information on child play that involved *make believe* and some parents struggle to recall this in their offspring. Examples of the child's play, if they can be recalled, are worth requesting from the informant in further probing questions; judgement can then be applied to deciding whether the example recalls refers to imaginative play. It is recommended for any clinician with limited experience of observing children behaving imaginatively to arrange for opportunities to do so.

Imitation (mimicking behaviour observed in someone else) should be enquired about at the same time as imaginative play because imitation might be mistaken for creative ability. Therefore, it is important to code separately *imitation*, repetitive, and particularly solitary play. Some play scenarios with peers may involve one child exerting dominance and leadership, instructing others in dress and behaviour (the 'director'). Children may share the process of making up the game—(as in multiple 'screenwriters').

Some families really do not seem to understand the meaning of questions about make believe play and tick the not known/not recalled response on the self-completion PPBS. Even at a very young age some children are good at concealing their play from grown-ups (Dunn 2004).

Bodily movements

Caregivers have little difficulty in describing unusual or unexpected bodily movements as listed in Box 3.4. It is unusual for informants who have not known the person as a child to be aware of these in the able individual.

Sensory differences

Parents and caregivers may only notice a few types of sensory difference and then mainly in more severely affected individuals. Current experience suggests that the adult patient interview is by far the best source of information on sensory differences (Chapter 8).

We still do not know to what extent these behaviours are specific to autism. An autism diagnosis should not be considered unless other behaviours characteristic of autism are also clearly identified.

Proximal sensory stimulation

Minor forms of repetitive touching behaviours, scratching, or sniffing, on their own have little if any clinical significance and, although not concealed from parents, may go unremarked upon because they are just part of what that child is. Anxiety levels may contribute to their frequency. Self-injury, unintended, can occur when anxiety levels are high and should not to be automatically taken as an indication of depression, although any associated *behaviour problems in childhood and adulthood* should be considered.

Parents may also recall striking examples of unusual responses to pain and temperature. A sensory checklist should include examples of these (Chapter 3).

Response to sounds

Parents are usually aware of unusual sensitivity to loud noises and to unusual ability to pick up quiet sounds in their offspring. They may also be aware of the rare and striking fascination some adults with autism have in particular sounds that they collect using digital or similar media. It is important to identify these as they may be important in supporting and making reasonable adjustments at work, and in home accommodation (Chapter 13).

Response to visual stimuli

Parents will give good accounts of these behaviours, which also tend to ameliorate with increasing age (in public settings at least). Partners and other adult intimates will also come to notice them as they spend more time relaxing with the affected person.

Routines and resistance to change

In general, parents and partners are aware of such behaviours, but they may not be as clear as to the extent the behaviours are enjoyed and sought by the individual, rather than performed compulsively. More difficult, sometimes, is to evaluate how intrusive and problematic such behaviours are. It may be helpful to ask whether day-to-day obligations and responsibilities are neglected, and whether such behaviours have put paid employment roles at jeopardy. Box 3.7 includes a checklist of the main examples, but is not exhaustive. Chapter 3 also includes definitions of ritual, routine, and of circumscribed interests.

Where seemingly specialized interests or 'fascinations' are identified, it is important to enquire whether these bring the person into contact with others socially, or have some other useful purpose. Case Study B (Chapter 2), provided a possible illustration of intolerance to change, as well as the example of a young adult who never joined in chit chat or conversation, which could be explored systematically in a developmental history.

Behaviour problems in childhood and adulthood

In the Past and Present Behaviour Schedule (PPBS), referred to previously, this section of the questionnaire, for carers to complete, is open-ended. They are asked to write down descriptions of the behaviours. It can be helpful to look at this part of the completed form first, before looking at the rest of the questionnaire, as it can reveal a great deal of information about the nature and significance of potential developmentally abnormal behaviours, and importantly of their developmental time course. For example, if the problems are listed as only occurring, or being problematic in recent (i.e. adult) years, it is almost certainly the case that we are not looking at a developmental disorder, but are instead dealing with something more familiar to the adult psychiatrist, an adult-onset mental or behavioural disorder, or possibly, what we term a personality disorder.

This section will also sometimes point up behaviours that may place others at risk, usually carers, but occasionally others, which do, of course, require follow-up investigation. It was suggested in Chapter 2, on awareness raising, to consider whether the person seems to need help in managing common-sense issues, including risks? People with autism are often vulnerable and at risk because of core autistic symptoms and coexisting mental health conditions, and for a significant number of autistic people, learning disabilities further increase their vulnerability (NICE, 2012). Any risk assessment of adults with autism should consider the risk of self-harm, in particular, the risk of suicide in people who are also depressed, but risk of harm to others also needs to be considered, particularly for family members and carers living at home where there may be significant incidents of challenging behaviour. This may not be uncovered unless questions are asked directly, which will be more straightforward when informants are interviewed separately.

Self-neglect may also come up at this point if not earlier in the interview. Neglect of physical health needs should be followed up, particularly if the patient has a record of disorganization and poor insight.

Seizures or other attacks

Epilepsy is a clearly established comorbidity in autism and should be routinely asked about.

Concluding remarks

The end of an interview with parents and carers is an opportunity to raise other concerns that may be more difficult to discuss with the patient also present. Concerns about risk to self and others, and safeguarding issues should be addressed here, unless covered already earlier in the interview, which may then need addressing elsewhere. Where it is looking likely that the diagnosis will be on the autism spectrum, it can be helpful to make a couple of general points about the need to discuss post-assessment support with carers and with the patient, once the outcome of the assessment is clear.

Chapter 8

Full assessment: interviewing the patient and autistic phenomenology

Introduction

The direct patient interview of an adult suspected of autism provides important opportunities to consider psychiatric comoribidities, which is covered in Chapter 10. It may also be a key opportunity to assess risk and consider its management. The NICE (2012) adult guideline group were particularly concerned about the risk of abuse and potential exploitation in people who may have autism. Where appropriate, the assessment of challenging behaviour includes not only the assessment of the behaviour itself, but of any underlying but unrecognised, physical or mental health disorders. The impact of the physical and social, including the home, environment will also need to be considered in the assessment of challenging behaviour, referred to in the previous chapter. Mindful of how adults with autism can attend narrowly and literally, to questions put to them, it is important to use the interview to ask directly but in a collaborative way, about risks.

The background to the approach to direct patient interviewing taken here derives from assessment principles used in the research and training instrument, the World Health Organization Schedules for Clinical Assessment in Neuropsychiatry (WHO SCAN; Wing et al. 1990; http://whoscan.org/). The approach taken is that of a semi-structured, investigator-rated assessment, as explained later in this chapter. Further background information and details on the SCAN interview are given in Appendix 3.

Interviewing procedures

It was decided to begin the interview with questions on attention, overactivity (seen in attention deficit hyperactivity disorder (ADHD)), and then on rigid and repetitive behaviours (RRBs), seen in autism. These seemed quite straightforward for patients to describe and refer to behaviours that patients might feel or that others have already observed in them, which are, in this sense, less 'private' and, perhaps, less stigmatizing. They also provide an opportunity to evaluate the extent to which the patient can recall and describe sufficiently clearly their childhood experiences, which are necessary for assessing whether autism has affected their child's development.

Questions are set out in groups that correspond to a key symptom (or 'item') of the condition (in these two examples, ADHD and RRB symptoms in autism). Further groups of questions then follow on sensory differences, social communication and interaction, and on social relationships. The latter two areas are more difficult for adults to describe. For convenience and to provide what could be vital collateral information on social development, appropriately reworded questions are included for informants where available to be interviewed.

For each set of symptoms or items, a definition of the abnormal form, which that behaviour takes, is placed alongside the suggested questions and probes. This approach, with these two essential parts—guidance on questioning and a glossary definition to guide rating of the absence, presence, severity of a symptom—dates back to the Present State Examination (Wing et al. 1974), from which SCAN was developed. Extended examples of the current Version 2.1 Interview and Glossary for symptoms of anxiety and depression (but not yet autism) can be downloaded at: http://whoscan.org/introduction/.

Table 8.1 lists the main subheadings to be covered in the assessment interview, and the underlying concept being evaluated by each set of questions. There are two parts—questions on rigid repetitive behaviours, and on social communication and social interaction.

Life-course and periods of time covered

The time period[1] to be covered in relation to neurodevelopmental symptoms will be lifelong, with ratings indicating whether any abnormally rated behaviour occurred in childhood only, in adulthood only, or in both periods of life. This approach has worked well in adult interviews on ADHD, and shows promise in interviews we have been conducting with adults, covering autism.

---

[1] For any reader unfamiliar with clinical psychiatry, questions about common and severe mental disorders will cover the past month before the interview, hence the term, 'present state examination'.

Table 8.1 Behaviours and symptoms to be covered when interviewing the patient to assess symptoms of autism spectrum disorder as experienced by an adult

Behaviours and symptoms (items)	Underlying concept being evaluated
Rigid repetitive behaviours	The extent to which the subject has a narrow range of interests/activities that are unusual, not shared or not particularly productive in encouraging social relationships or a career. How far his/her activities are repetitive (e.g. collecting unnecessary copies of the same object).
Restricted, circumscribed interests	
Routines, rituals	
Repetitive behaviours	
Rigidity	The extent to which rigidity is a characteristic—to the degree that the subject has difficulty in coping with unexpected change. That is, the extent to which (s)he is a slave to a routine or to some ritual.
Sensory differences	The extent to which over- or under-sensitivity and pre-occupation with differences in sensory experiences interfere with important activities, such as work, rest, and leisure, and the ability to interact with others.
Problems with social communication and social interaction	The extent to which the respondent shows an interest in and curiosity about the life of key others, which goes beyond their shared activities and interests, and is able to engage in informal social conversation and to pick up (or gauge) how the other person feels from observing their non-verbal reactions and, in turn, is able to show their own feelings through non-verbal self-expression.
Social interest and intuition	
Social conversation	
Non-verbal communication (recognition and expression)	
Social relationships	The extent to which the respondent is able to engage and participate in relationships with family, close others, and friends.

Rigid repetitive behaviours

Case Study E in Chapter 2 described an adult with fixed habits and rituals, which could be evaluated through the developmental history or by an interview with the patient. The following fairly general questions are taken from the original interview guide referenced above. If replies to these questions do not elicit any evidence of behaviours or symptoms of this kind, and if there is no other information pointing to RRBs, the interview should move onto the next section, covering social communication and social interaction:

> Tell me about your hobbies/special interests?
> How much time do you spend on these?
> Do you have any collections? (Tell me about them.)
> Do you share this interest with anyone? (Belong to any clubs/societies)
> How organized a person are you? Are there things you like to do a certain way or to a set routine?
> - Have you ever had set routines?
> - What happens when you can't do things in the way you would like (or when you have to change your plans)?
>
> Some people seem to be unusually sensitive (or insensitive) to certain sensations. For example, they are very aware of specific sounds, smells, textures?
> - Are you affected in this way?

Note, in the last example but one, above, that the main question wording ('How organized are you…?') is followed by several alternative probes. The style of interviewing is very much intended to proceed in this flexible way, the additional probes being asked only if the initial question has not elicited any clear information. The experienced interviewer, who has a clear mental concept of the symptom that is being assessed, will be able to adapt the wording of such probe questions to the level of understanding and language development of the interview respondent (or patient). While this may risk introducing some element of interviewer variability (and arguable loss of reliability) into the interview process, it is believed that validity is improved through better understanding and communication between interviewer and respondent.

More specific probes on rigid repetitive behaviours with brief examples of glossary definitions

Examples of some of the questions and follow-up probes for inflexible behaviours follow here, which may be helpful if the above questions generate potentially positive responses, or if it is unclear from the responses whether the symptoms or behaviours are present, or are clinically significant at any time in childhood or currently.

Restricted, circumscribed interests

- Is this [interest] something you do on your own or does it involve other people? (Does it mean that you meet or talk to others with the same interest?)
- How many people do you talk to about your interest?
- How has your interest developed over time? Has it extended into work or other roles?

Excerpt from corresponding definition for this symptom:

> ... [an] interest that is abnormally intense in its focus or unusual in its content and use, is not shared with others, is restricted in its extent and has little practical application ...

Routines, rituals

Do you have routines in the way you organize your life from day to day?

Do you like to vary what you wear or do you tend to stick to the same kind of clothes?

Excerpt from corresponding definition of this symptom:

> A *routine*—a sequence of actions regularly followed in the same, particular order ...
>
> A *ritual*—a series of actions that hold some additional, higher significance for the person performing them. Examples are an unusually elaborate way of dressing ...

Repetitive behaviours

How much does it seem to take up time for more important things, duties, obligations, work?

How has it developed over time?

Excerpt from corresponding definition for this symptom:

> Actions or sequences of behaviour that are relatively rapidly repeated in a manner that does not appear to have a functional utility ...

Rigidity

Do you like to live your life by clear rules?

How flexible are you in coping with change, caused by people who are close (your friends, family, partner, children)?

Excerpt from corresponding definition for this symptom:

The lack of mental flexibility—either in the abnormal adherence to rules, or difficulty experienced with other minor changes...

Sensory differences

How sensitive is your hearing? Are there noises that you can't stand? Or sounds you like listening to repeatedly?

What about smells—do you have a good sense of smell? Do certain smells bother or alarm you?

Excerpt from corresponding definition for this symptom:

Experiencing hypo/hyper-sensitivity to a sensory modality, e.g. indifference to pain/temperature, an adverse response to everyday sounds; seeking/avoiding sensations—so that the person avoids or seeks an area or activity...

Problems with social communication and social interaction

The following fairly general questions on social communication and interaction are taken from the training interview guide, referred to in Appendix 3, which follows the same approach. If replies to these questions do not elicit any evidence of this kind of problem behaviour, or difficulties in engaging in social communication and social interaction, and if there is no other information pointing to such difficulties, the interviewer can move onto the next part of the assessment process.

Questions on social communication

How chatty do you think you are? Do you enjoy chatting?

- How easy is it to respond when someone else talks to you?
- How able are you to make small talk?
- Do you ever say too much and not know when to stop?
- Do others comment on how you talk (that you say too much/too little)?

Are you the sort of person who shows your feelings? For example, are you an affectionate person?
- How do you show your affection?
- What do you do if someone close to you tries to hug you?

Can you show me a happy face?
- What kinds of things make you happy?
- How would you describe the feeling of being happy to someone who has never felt happy?

What about a sad face—look sad.
- What kind of things makes you depressed?
- How would you describe the feeling of being depressed to someone who has never felt depressed?

What about an anxious face?
- What kind of things makes you anxious?
- How would you describe the feeling of being anxious to someone who has never felt anxious?

When you first went to school, did other people have any difficulty in understanding what you said?

When you were a child, did people ever comment on the way you spoke? Compared to the other children around you, were you any different?

Questions on relationship functioning

Tell me about your friends? (List names and check ages.)
- How long have you known them.
- Tell me about your friends at school/college/work. (Check whether peers/staff.)

Tell me about the sort of things you like doing together?
- How often do you see them?

Do you ever feel lonely?
- Tell me about the sort of things you can do to make yourself feel better.

What does being a friend mean to you?

Tell me about a friend compared with someone you just meet at work/college.
- How easy is it for you to make friends (and to keep them)?

Do you have a boyfriend/girlfriend? (Note the name.)
- How long have you been together?
- How do you know she is your boyfriend/girlfriend?

More specific probes on social communication and social interaction with brief examples of glossary definitions

A few more examples of some of the questions follow here, which expand on the above, in more detail and which may be helpful in clarifying the clinical significance of the patient's initial responses.

Social conversation, interest in others and social intuition

Do you like the informal, social gossip side of such [informal] gatherings? Or do you think it is unnecessary, a waste of time, or disapprove of it, or find it uncomfortable?

Short excerpt from corresponding definition for this symptom:

Social curiosity refers to the person's innate desire to discover other people's experiences and feelings, as well as tell others about their own experiences and feelings ... [not just a scientific like curiosity]

Social intuitiveness refers to the ability to appreciate what the other person is thinking and feeling, without having to consciously work it out ...

Non-verbal communication (recognition and expression)

When you are talking to people, how good are you at recognizing when they are starting to get bored?

How do you work out how they are feeling?

Short excerpt from corresponding glossary definition for this symptom:

The person's ability to read and respond to the non-verbal communication of other people ...

Social relationships

What are your friends interested in? What do they like doing?

Do you share things with them about your personal life? Do you know what is happening in their personal lives?

Short excerpt from corresponding glossary definition for this symptom:

The ability to form and maintain peer relationships is an innate skill, for many, which matures with the person ...

Further procedural steps and conclusions

As in a thorough clinical 'work-up', or medical 'detailing', it is important to record verbatim examples of the words and phrases patients use to describe their experiences, in relation to these behaviours. A colleague examining the record will then be able to judge its veracity and any changes that might emerge in a follow-up interview, which might take place many years subsequently, possibly signalling improved functioning. This may also assist research in the future; there is a dearth of such descriptive material on the experience of autism in adulthood, and most of it is spontaneously expressed, which although inherently extremely valuable, lacks the systematic structured approach outlined here.

It is a standard procedure to rate insight into difficulties. This will be useful and important in considering post-diagnostic support, training, care, and follow-up.

Interference with activities due to each major group of symptoms is also rated. A record of the interviewer's judgement of interference should also be made, and will be important in deciding what post-diagnostic input is warranted. As has been said several times in this book, the need to diagnose and support adults on the autism spectrum depends crucially on this (and is an explicit part of the DSM-5 criteria for Autism Spectrum Disorder).

During the interview there will have been numerous opportunities to observe the patient, and the manner in which they communicate and interact with you, the interviewer, and others, such as carers who they may have chosen to invite to an assessment (or staff observing the patient in a care setting). In the next chapter we will explore how to elicit, describe, and rate such observations directly.

Acknowledgements

Most of the material in this chapter has been developed jointly with Dr Tom Berney of the University of Newcastle and Dr Peter Carpenter, Bristol, UK, supported by an international collaborative group with expertise in the assessment of adult psychopathology, who serve as advisers on the World Health Organization Schedules for Clinical Assessment in Neuropsychiatry (SCAN: http://whoscan.org/).

Chapter 9

Full assessment: direct observation and the signs of autism

Background

As has been mentioned on many occasions already in this book, traditionally, the diagnosis of autism has rested on direct or informant conveyed observation of the child (and in recent years, the adult who has not already been diagnosed in childhood). In adulthood opportunities for direct observation are often limited to the traditional short consultation, much of which is artificially dominated by direct questioning, which may mask the patient's normal day-to-day style of communication. This is also true of public health surveys, where no more than a short interview with the survey respondent will be acceptable. Methods have been developed, in child autism research, for formalizing the assessment of observations of the child's communication with caregivers and with others. This has some value, but also some limitation in the adult context.

A particular limitation of the observational approach may apply in the context of comorbidity and, since psychiatric comorbidity is very likely to be more common in the patients adult psychiatrists are seeing, this issue will be addressed both here and in Chapter 10, on comorbidity assessment.

In this chapter suggestions will be included on how to code, in a fairly simple and time-efficient way, key observable aspects of non-verbal communication. There will be times when a more detailed systematic assessment of observed behaviour is called for, particularly when the diagnosis is unclear. Ideally, this should be performed with administration of a formal evaluation of social communication and reciprocal social interaction, which can be performed by a trained assistant as part of a general evaluation. Finally, as in the tradition of psychopathology assessment, just covered in the previous chapter, reference will be made to descriptions of striking and more severe variations from neurotypical behaviour, sometimes seen in autism in adulthood, which forms part of the overall approach to assessment.

The place of direct observation in adult psychiatry and in the psychiatry of autism

Before the development of modern psychiatry and psychopathology, particularly from the nineteenth century onwards, it seems reasonable to assume, with rare and largely unrecorded exceptions, that the assessment of the mental state was based on observation of behaviour and occasionally on publicly accessible accounts of what patients wrote or said about it. The modern era has seen this approach largely replaced, in the verbally able and fluent adult, by the development of skilfully devised interview techniques, as set out in Chapter 8. Observation has perhaps been neglected (except in the psychiatry of intellectual disability, where few patients are capable of talking about their experiences).

There is some empirical justification for that neglect of observation, within adult mental health. Assessments of the reliability of direct observations of patients by doctors observing them together (or independently in succession to one another) were discouraging. The observations covered the areas of speech (and language), mood, and other aspects of behaviour.[1] A particular challenge is the question as to how reliable and valid observations of variations in modes of communication in autism are, in the context of severe mental illness.[2] This will be discussed further in the Chapter 10, 'Comorbidity assessments'. Only one approach to measuring observed

---

[1] The SCAN interview provides a comprehensive list of such observations, grouped in relation to all the major domains of psychopathology (Wing et al. 1990; http://whoscan.org/). Consideration was given to removing these observational sections from the SCAN, during an international meeting of SCAN advisers, under WHO auspices, in the 1980s. They were retained because observation of the patient still held currency in the training of psychiatrists. This seems to continue unquestioned; it may be that in certain contexts, such as intensive care and acute and crisis psychiatry, this is a sensible policy.

[2] As an adult psychiatrist, viewing observation in psychiatry with some scepticism, the 'discovery' of the considerable value of observation in autism was a surprise. Training in the Autism Diagnostic Observation Schedule (ADOS; Lord et al. 2002), leads to a re-evaluation of the value of direct observation. The search for a survey measure of autism in adulthood showed that developmental histories could not be gathered on thousands of survey respondents. Training in this form of observational approach should be part of the specialist training of both child and adult psychiatrists.

behaviour, in mentally ill patients, seemed to have acceptable reliability and that required the systematic rating of input of caregivers, such as careworkers and nurses, observing the patient regularly if not daily over a period of 1 month (Wykes and Sturt, 1986). Official classification systems also largely abandoned the requirement to include such observations, although in the latest iteration of the DSM this shows signs of returning in relation to the diagnosis of depression.[3]

Essentials of effective observation of behaviour

In adulthood, opportunities for direct observation are often limited to the traditional short consultation, much of which is artificially dominated by direct questioning, which may mask the patient's normal day-to-day style of communication. This is also true of public health surveys, where no more than a short interview with the survey respondent will be acceptable. Both are also now dominated by the interviewer's need to enter data via a keyboard while viewing a monitor or screen and, therefore, not looking at how the patient is responding to the flow of the interview. A clear requirement of the ADOS procedure is that specific tasks are included, in which the interviewer acts as an observer, pausing from recording notes or ratings. For most psychiatrists this may require a departure from customary ways of working. Later in this chapter a series of key observational headings are described—eye gaze, gesture, facial expression, vocal intonation.

Short overview of the Autism Diagnostic Observation Schedule (ADOS)

Methods have been developed in child autism research for formalizing the assessment of observations of the child's communication, with caregivers, peers, and others. Like many of the assessment approaches described in this book, the ADOS was developed for research purposes, but also for use in clinical settings and, therefore, as part of more specialized training. Arguably all clinical staff based in adult diagnostic service should receive

---

[3] A Pubmed search linking the mesh terms gestural communication and mental disorder found a few studies on autism, two on schizophrenia, e.g. (White et al. 2016) and none on depression, with dementia receiving some attention. Clearly, research on gestural communication in psychiatry has been surprisingly neglected, although the topic seemed to hold promise in the post-World War II years (Argyle, 1978).

training in its use. ADOS Module 4 (ADOS-4) was designed for the older child and younger adult.[4] When the author began to use Module 4, it had undergone very little testing or further development, and had hardly been used regularly on older adults. Further details of its evaluation in adult populations are set out in Appendix 4.

The ADOS-4 provides a direct face-to-face assessment of current respondent behaviour suitable for adults undergoing assessment for an autistic disorder (Lord et al. 2002). It covers communication, reciprocal social interaction and, in a limited way, restricted and repetitive behaviours. It consists of various tests comprising set situations (termed '*presses*') that enable the evaluation of communication, reciprocal social interaction, creativity, imagination, and stereotyped behaviour and restricted interests. In the child versions, play materials are used to elicit behaviours that are observed and rated according to specific guidance; some elements of this approach are retained in Module 4. Respondents are also asked about their knowledge and understanding of social relationships, emotions, and daily living responsibilities.

Examples of techniques used in the ADOS to help generate respondent communication

What follows is a selection of some of the techniques used to help to bring out behaviours that may be relevant to autism. There are detailed manuals describing the method in full (Lord et al. 2002).

Adults with autism may find it difficult to give an extended account of a past event in which they have participated. They will just mention the barest details or give too full an account that loses sight of what their audience needs to hear. They will answer any questions on specific facts—so direct questions are easier for them to respond to. This characteristic probably reflects their difficulty in engaging in sociable discussion. In ADOS Module 4 this is addressed under the heading 'Conversation and Reporting'. The examiner observes and notes the extent to which the respondent is able to talk about a routine and non-routine event while making use of non-verbal signals (as listed earlier). Immediately after completing the interview, the examiner completes various ratings, including a rating of how what the

---

[4] There are four ADOS modules, numbered 1–4; recently a fifth module for toddlers has been added. Each module corresponds to a particular age and stage of development. Module 1 is suitable for pre-verbal children, which we have used with a few adaptations to assess non-verbal adults (Brugha et al. 2016). Modules 2 and 3 cover intermediate stages of verbally able childhood.

respondent says elaborates on comments by the interviewer. It reflects to and fro changes in the direction of the conversation, arising from what each person says. At the same time the interviewer makes written notes of various aspects of gesture, expression, use of gaze, etc. Respondents are also asked to comment on a detailed photograph, describing the scene depicted in it. The spontaneous use of language is noted, as it is also as respondents look through a picture story book (chosen to be of likely interest to all age groups). A specific method is also used to elicit gesture—or, at least, nonverbal ways of demonstrating a task. The task suggested is a demonstration of tooth brushing.

Adaptation of observational methods to the autism clinical evaluation setting—the example of gesture

In the clinic, in situations in which the ADOS is not being formally rated, for example in a short and necessarily rapid triage evaluation (Table 6.2), similar techniques are followed, or they are adapted.[5] For example, in order to elicit gesture (where it has not occurred spontaneously), one first notes whether the patient's hands and arms are observable or hidden, and whether they are free (the patient may be clutching paperwork or personal belongings). Hands need to be free to permit gesture to occur freely—if necessary, the patient is asked to put down, or put away, any object that is obstructing this. At some point during the interview the patient will be asked to talk to the examiner about something they like to do with their hands, such as grooming their pet, planting a shrub, preparing a preferred dish, painting a toy model. Most adults, quite unconsciously, use gesture that is descriptive or informational in some sense, when talking about something like this. In autism, gesture may be present, but it is likely to be less complex in its expression than in the neurotypical adult. Adults also use gesture by way of emphasis, particularly when talking about something quite exciting or emotional, so it is important to encourage opportunities for these things to happen. Direct questions about emotions (adapting the mental state interview), relationships, and work, all covered in a conventional psychiatric assessment, also provide opportunities to observe. However, it is important to record those observations as they occur—sometimes they may be more important than what the patient says.

---

[5] In the formal research using the ADOS, led by the author, all of the instructions in the ADOS manual are followed precisely.

> **Box 9.1 Observations of non-verbal communication**
>
> - *Gaze*: skilful and reflective or fixed, staring, looking at objects in the room, glancing fleetingly?
> - *Gesture*: emotional, emphatic, instrumental, informational, descriptive; absent or occasional use only, self-conscious, and manneristic?
> - *Facial expression*; fixed or variable, reflective of what is talked about, informative?
> - *Vocal intonation*: monotonous or varied, unusual volume (too loud or quiet), odd, or unusual for age (child-like in an adult when there are no children present)?

Box 9.1 sets out techniques found to be useful and which can easily be melded into a short consultation. Ask yourself how much, if ever, do you use these techniques? If not, one suggestion might be to print out Box 9.2, and have it ready for the next consultation with a patient who seems to display some of the alerting characteristics of possible autism (Chapter 2).

Observing non-verbal signs and communication

Surprisingly little research on non-verbal communication in mental illness has been carried out since the topic was reviewed in the late 1970s (Argyle, 1978). A rare exception has recently been shown that people with schizophrenia can have difficulties in interpreting social cues (White et al. 2016).

Box 9.1 lists the key non-verbal communication channels that are essential to observe and record in any consultation, particularly a first contact. There are growing views that there are gender variations in these, within autism, such that autism may be more easily missed in women if based only on these kinds of observations (see earlier chapters). In the next chapter, differences attributable to other mental and behavioural disorders will also need to be considered.

A further list of more striking and perhaps, more severe forms of abnormal non-verbal communication (seen in long-term adult care settings) can be found later in this chapter in Box 9.6 showing examples of lack of non-verbal communication.

Box 9.2 Principles to follow in generating observations of social interaction

- Observe (stop listening for a moment—just look and take it all in—vocal intonation, gaze, gesture, variation in facial expression).
- Make a brief reminder note immediately of what you observe; *don't wait*; you may forget.
- Vary your behaviour.
- Make it easy by asking direct questions.
- Make it challenging by saying nothing, passing comments, pausing without explanation, and not asking questions (no matter how tempting to do so).
- Make it different by seeing the patient with others they know and seeing the patient alone.
- Change your demeanour from cheerful to stern, from puzzled and perplexed to controlling and inflexible.
- Encourage talk and greater non-verbal expression by referring to a known interest or fascination of the patient, and show some interest.
- Test sociability by *interrupting* with something you find interesting, and watch to see if the respondent can accept and show some effort at a similar interest or is troubled by the interruption.
- Abandon your familiar comfortable questioning and information gathering professional style for at least part of the consultation.

Gaze

The key to abnormal use of eye gaze in the adult with autism is a complete lack of 'natural' gaze, i.e. a lack of gaze that seems to flow automatically, without the person needing to think consciously about what they are doing (and 'giving messages with the eyes', a phrase used by Lorna Wing). Looking at you and not doing so (but not 'knowing', or being aware, (s)he is doing so). Looking when you are talking to them. Looking less when they are talking to you. Some very anxious patients begin by hardly looking at the interviewer, but gradually learn to relax and use gaze more normally as the consultation proceeds.

Some patients stare at objects and only occasionally look at the interviewer, which is a possible suggestion of autism. If autism has been suspected since childhood (or diagnosed officially), the patient may have been taught strategies for dealing with problems with eye gaze, such as gaze fixation. The person they are communicating with may feel that they are being stared at. One technique is the advice [to the patient] to look at the other person's nose or mouth, if looking at their eyes proves too difficult or, indeed, painful. Another common form of advice is, if in doubt, to look down (which is less threatening). During a prolonged consultation, one observes that these initially quite effective strategies break down. Again, this is why it is important to have time for observation.

Gesture

It is almost impossible to suppress gesture. Great actors who have portrayed autism (or 'Asperger syndrome') convincingly, have accounted how difficult and tiring it is to consciously suppress gesture.

We tend to be unaware of our own gesture. Gesture varies enormously in its amount and expressiveness, from person to person, and probably varies a good deal between cultures. When assessing a young adult, with the help of both parents in attendance, one will also use gesture far more than the other. When this is pointed out to the family, they often seem to hear this news as though they were never aware of it (siblings perhaps excepted).

We use gesture to convey emphasis (recalling Khrushchev removing his shoe to pound the table at the United Nations). We also use gesture to convey symbolically what we feel strongly about. Primates also use gesture. There are relatively few hard and fast, or universal rules about what particular gestures mean. We react more strongly to others who use gesture in communication. This may be one of the reasons why it can be so easy to lose interest in listening to someone on the spectrum—not because what they are saying isn't interesting, but rather, because it is not backed up with gesture (and other non-verbal cues). Head nodding and shaking, hand clapping and handshaking, are all a form of gesture, and pointing is possibly the first gesture we learn to use (and following others who are pointing).

If there is a 'clinical test' that sometimes seems to work in autism, it is the quality (and willingness to proffer it) of a handshake. Like gaze, it just seems very natural and unselfconscious, when typical, and more like something learnt, and not learnt well, when given by a person on the spectrum. (This is also another opportunity to observe the engagement of eyes that conventionally accompanies a hand shake, or a 'hi five!' greeting). Another is that when the autistic patient finally leaves the consulting room, they rarely look back to glance at you, one final time, but their carers usually do. Hence, perhaps, the unfair, but understandable use of the term 'cold', to describe people on the spectrum.

Facial expression

Darwin wrote a book on the subject of non-verbal expression, devoting much time to facial expression and the anatomical structure of the muscles underlying it (Darwin, 1873). Michael Argyle took up the subject a century later stating that 'the face is the most important non-verbal channel' (Argyle, 1987).

Like all forms of non-verbal communication, facial expression varies enormously between people. We all interact with people who have none or almost no variation in facial expression, and hardly seem aware of it, unless we consciously alert ourselves to do so. Expression can also be learnt and taught quite convincingly, until there is some departure from predictable conventional scripts. This is why the assessment needs to be challenging. Are there expressions of spontaneous pleasure, anxiety, and sadness—these will only happen if there are opportunities. Traps to the unwary clinician include the fixed 'grimace', which seems to be a smile, until you ask yourself is there any other expression other than a neutral face. Another possible trap is Parkinsonism, especially if medicated.

Expression can be 'acted', of course. However, many patients on the autism spectrum, when asked to put on a face corresponding to sadness or fear, refuse to do so, claiming they cannot do so. Able women on the spectrum may be better able to 'fake normal' (a term they use to describe imitation used in communicating with others who do not know of their difficulties). They may also seem to exaggerate expressions (perhaps they have learnt this—at present we do not know). Particularly difficult seems to be to integrate facial expression with gaze and gesture, for which there are specific codes on the ADOS.

Vocal intonation

You really have to be very conscious of vocal intonation to notice abnormalities in it, unless you realize it at the very first utterance by the patient or if the voice is so quiet that you have to ask the patient to repeat what they say. Classically, the voice in autism sounds like it is generated by a computer programme—monotonous and almost mechanical sounding. Sometimes, it only dawns on the clinician, when they are meeting with a parent or informant, and the patient—the former showing natural vocal intonation, emphasis, change in pitch, or being too fast or too slow.

Have you ever felt a patient in your consultation room was talking so loud that you felt people in the next room could hear what (s)he was saying? Did you feel awkward, embarrassed, or concerned? Did you think of autism?[6]

---

[6] Other possible explanations could be poor hearing, or a person living with someone who has poor hearing and who has to raise their voice to be heard.

> **Box 9.3 Observations of social communication**
>
> - Does (s)he show curiosity, ask for information not strictly part of the consultation?
> - Is talk about emotional topics accompanied by emotional expression, such as tearfulness, signs of fear, arousal, enjoyment?
> - If there is a third party present does the patient glance at the other person from time to time or behave as if they are not there?
> - How is attention maintained? Do the patient's responses reflect your comments or only respond to direct questions or personal pre-occupations
> - Does (s)he seem to know when they have spoken too long about a topic, i.e. that it's time to stop?
> - Can (s)he talk reflecting creative thinking, or does it always seem to refer to facts and prepared topics?
> - Does (s)he pause sometimes to check that what they are saying is relevant and employ eye gaze to reflect this enquiry?

Observing social communication

Box 9.3 lists some of the observations one can make of styles of social communication. Take the time to make these observations in patients you are confident are not autistic, and then in someone who is clearly judged to be significantly affected on the autism spectrum. You can also try to make these sorts of observations in day-to-day settings outside the consulting room.

Observations of more striking and unusual behaviours that may be associated with autism

As in the tradition of psychopathology assessment covered in the previous chapter, reference should be made to descriptions of striking and more severe variations from neurotypical behaviour, sometimes seen in autism in adulthood, which forms part of the overall assessment.[7]

---

[7] Many of these types of observable behaviour are included in the current WHO SCAN interview.

Catatonia in autism

Before listing these observations, mention needs to be given to the topic of catatonia. Traditionally, catatonia was presumed to be part of schizophrenia (World Health Organization, 1993). It is still commonly seen in low and middle-income country (LMIC) rural societies.[8] However, most psychiatrists seeing adults in the most developed, high-income countries, have either never seen catatonia, or on only one or two occasions. Observable features of catatonia recorded in the SCAN are listed in an adapted form in Box 9.4. It is striking now, looking at these features, to think how so many of them could be observed in more severely disabled autistic adults. Examples that stand out in Box 9.4 are negativism, hesitation, echopraxia, opposition, jerkiness, freezing, complex mannerisms, adoption of odd postures, stereotypies.

On observing catatonic posturing and hesitation in a young man, on an inpatient unit in the 1990s (it had not been mentioned in the written case notes), Dr Wing offered to advise. She enquired if catatonia been considered to be part of the patient's autism (that had been diagnosed)? Several cases have been seen since, none of whom have shown positive psychotic symptoms. Dr Amita Shah who co-authored a paper on this topic with Dr Lorna Wing (Wing and Shah, 2000) was able to see and advise helpfully on the first of these patients. Catatonia associated with autism is now a specific code in DSM-5.

Other behaviours observed particularly in long-term care settings

The additional observations listed in Box 9.5 may also prove useful in observing patients in long-term care or in homeless settings, such as adults who are sleeping rough, people begging in the street. These are not behaviours that are particularly characteristic of autism, but if seen in a clinical setting the possibility of autism, with or without some element of intellectual disability, should be given some consideration unless it has already been ruled out.

The SCAN interview, in its current form, also includes ratings of observations of lack of non-verbal communication (adapted in Box 9.6), the commoner and less severe forms of which are discussed earlier in this chapter. These observations should also raise the question of possible autism spectrum disorder. Some indication of the severity of the behaviour can also be described.

---

[8] Colleagues who began their training in rural India mention this often.

Box 9.4 Features of catatonic behaviour, which are now thought to occur occasionally in the presence of autism (DSM-5)

Negativism
Patient does that opposite to what is asked by the examiner.

Hesitation (ambitendence)
Patient is unable to complete a movement, for example, passing through a door (advances, withdraws, advances again, begins to take examiners hand then withdraws, etc.)

Forced grasping
Takes hand repeatedly. Does so when asked not to by the examiner.

Echopraxia
Echolalia, imitates movements, repeats phrases.

Flexibilitas cerea
Lead pipe rigidity. Arms remain where placed for 15 seconds or more. Distinguish from resistance.

Opposition
Movement in any direction is countered by equal resistance in the opposite direction.

Jerkiness
Lack of smoothness of voluntary movements for 15 seconds or more.

Freezing
Limb remains in one position during voluntary movement.

Automatic obedience
Fingertip pressure on any part of the body produces movement in that direction.

Complex mannerisms
Odd stylized and idiosyncratic movements or actions, e.g. tapping foot four times before entering a doorway.

Posturing

Odd postures of parts of body, e.g. 'Balinese dancer' posture of hands and fingers (the posture adopted may imitate a more familiar contemporary style).

Simple stereotypies

Repetitive movements. Rocking, rubbing, nodding, swaying, twisting objects, tapping, feeling surfaces.

Source: data from *Arch Gen Psychiatry*, 47(6), Wing JK, Babor TT, Brugha TT, et al., SCAN: Schedules for Clinical Assessment in Neuropsychiatry, pp. 589–593, Copyright 1990, *American Medical Association; Diagnostic and Statistical Manual of Mental Disorders*, Fifth Edition, Copyright 2013, American Psychiatric Association.

Box 9.5 Other behaviours rarely seen that may occur more often in long-term care and institutional settings, which although not characteristic of autism should raise the question of whether autism is present and unrecognized

Mannerisms

Odd stylized and idiosyncratic movements or actions, e.g. tapping foot four times before entering a doorway.

Odd behaviours

Sniffing at other people. Tip toe walking (more than just walking with a bounce in the street).

Stereotyped behaviours

Repetitive movements. Rocking, rubbing, nodding, swaying, twisting objects, tapping, feeling surfaces.

Odd or inappropriate appearance

Odd clothes, ornaments, etc. Would stand out in a social group because of markedly inappropriate appearance.

Embarrassing behaviour

Making sexual advances, loss of social restraint, e.g. scratches genitals, passes loud flatus, etc.

Bizarre behaviour

Special ornaments or clothes with idiosyncratic meanings. Make-up bizarrely applied. Appearance grossly eccentric and embarrassing.

Self-neglect

Clothes inadequate for warmth and protection, irrespective of whether odd or embarrassing. Unkempt. Dirty. Smelly. Unshaven.

Neglect of health care

Inadequate diet. Ignores need for shelter. Grossly neglects physical disabilities or diseases, or attention to dental hygiene—caries, ill-fitting dentures, does not use dentures.

Personal hygiene and habits

Spits, smears, eats rubbish.

Self-injury

Head banging, picking sores, biting self, etc.

Neglect of common dangers

Does not understand common dangers, e.g. wanders across busy roads, cannot be trusted with gas taps, electric fires, etc.

Hoarding objects

Collection of old newspapers or useless objects.

Inane giggling or inappropriate laughter

Must be non-congruent with social or emotional context.

Behaviour associated with single interest

The interest must exclude or modify almost every other form of activity so that it appears markedly odd.

Box 9.6 Further observational descriptions: lack of non-verbal communication

Negative posture

In the milder form there is passive aversion, for example, the eyes are closed, posture is hunched, head bowed, and in the more severe form, the behaviour suggests active aversion, with the head turned away, so that the patient avoids eye contact, or the back is turned.

Gesture

In its milder form there is little use of gesture to accompany speech or illustrate meaning, and in the more severe form there is virtually no use of gesture of any kind.

Facial expression

In the milder form there is little change in expression to accompany or illustrate meaning or feeling. When more severe there is a virtually expressionless face that gives no clue to the patient's inner thoughts or feelings.

Expression in the voice

In its lesser form the voice changes little in expression with change of topic, and in its more severe form the voice is monotonous and expressionless throughout all speech.

Eye-contact

In its milder form eye contact is used unskilfully, for example the patient stares or gives wrong cue. In its more clinically significant form the patient makes almost no eye contact at all or it is only inappropriate.

Source: data from *Arch Gen Psychiatry*, 47(6), Wing JK, Babor TT, Brugha TT, et al., SCAN: Schedules for Clinical Assessment in Neuropsychiatry, pp. 589–593, Copyright 1990, American Medical Association.

It is interesting to note that these kinds of observations (Box 9.6) may well have been pointed out and taught to many adult psychiatrists, in training, particularly when working in either intensive or long-term care settings, although the idea that autism might explain these observations may hardly ever have been mentioned.

Possible limitations of observations of behaviour

A particular limitation may apply to reliance on observation in assessing autism, this being in the context of comorbidity, in particular. Since psychiatric comorbidity is very likely to be commoner in the patients adult psychiatrists are seeing in their clinical work, this issue will be addressed in the next chapter (Chapter 10) on comorbidity assessment. We will then look at additional assessments that may be of value in confirmed and in more severe cases of autism, focusing on psychological and social functioning within the adult world (Chapter 11), identifying factors of importance, in identifying needs, including issues of vulnerability and risk, and in developing a longer-term support and or care plan (Part III).

Chapter 10

Comorbidity assessment

Background

Adult psychiatrists have a particular opportunity to undertake the assessment and management of autism, and its associated psychiatric comorbidities, in a way that other professions in medicine would have greater difficulty with. There is growing awareness that autism can complicate adult mental disorder, can be overlooked, and that patients and their families welcome, and hugely appreciate, psychiatrists who are competent and confident in dealing with it.

It might be argued by general psychiatrists that they are not specialists, and, even if interested, cannot always become specialists in autism. Neither can they overlook a condition that has a significant impact on behaviour, perception, and emotional functioning in 1% of the adult population and quite possibly in 4% of their patients. Furthermore, in the UK, duties in law are constantly evolving and autism is increasingly contributing to that framework.

Expectations in law including mental capacity

In England there are expectations in law in two areas, in particular, the *restriction of liberty* and the *assessment of mental capacity*. Psychiatrists do not act alone in either of these areas of responsibility, but they have statutory roles, working alongside other professionals, both because of their knowledge and their assessment expertise in relation to behaviour and its possible causes. Accordingly, in restricting the freedom of certain adults, under particular circumstances, at specific times, the quality of the psychiatric assessment, including a risk assessment, is crucial to the proper delivery of their responsibilities (Berney et al. 2014). They are also expected to have basic competencies, and as trainers, to oversee the achievement of these competencies by less experienced doctors, working with them. Patients are entitled under law to reasonable adjustments being made taking account of disabilities affecting them and psychiatrists have a role in pointing these out although not in ensuring that others act on their advice. This topic is discussed further at the end of Chapter 12.

The topic of duties in relation to reasonable adjustments to autism is also relevant to many other individuals, and organizations, in our society, which will be covered in Part III of this volume. Psychiatrists (and doctors) also have duties to make reasonable adjustments for autism itself, and this places expectations on them to have the necessary knowledge and understanding to be able to do so. These expectations may not apply in all jurisdictions around the world, yet. However, one hopes that they will be, eventually, as interpretation of human rights extends into this area.

Caveats and key terms

It is perhaps understandable that some hard pressed colleagues in adult psychiatry, picking up this book for the first time, will be tempted to go straight to this chapter, on the topic of comorbidity assessment. Unless the reader has already covered elsewhere in training the background and assessment topics, set out in the first nine chapters of this book, this would be akin to entering clinical medicine with almost no knowledge of anatomy, physiology, pathology, and unguided, at that.

First, we will look at issues and challenges underlying comorbidity assessment, including potential confusion arising from words or terms that have long been with us in psychiatry, such as 'psychosis' and 'autism', misconceptions about premorbid functioning, and normal and abnormal development, from birth onwards, and common misdiagnoses. We will then unpick what we mean by course and development, common sources of under-recognition and misdiagnosis, including masking by other disorders, and the strengths and limitations of the range of approaches that can be taken in assessment. Important specific pathognomonic symptoms and comorbid disorders will then be covered, including those pertaining to ADHD, anxiety, obsessive compulsive disorder, depression, intellectual disability, epilepsy, and psychosis.

Issues and challenges in mental disorder and autism comorbidity assessment

A source of confusion may arise from the historical usage in psychiatry of the terms psychosis and autism (and psychopathy). Colman defines autism as 'a pathological self-absorption and preoccupation with the self to the exclusion of the outside world' (Colman 2001). Bleuler used the term in his writings on what we still call schizophrenia to refer to a symptom (not a syndrome). These are descriptive usages.

As discussed in Chapter 1, Kanner, who wrote the first textbook of child psychiatry, coined the term in his classic description of a small series of children with autism (Kanner 1943) under the title 'autistic disturbances of affective contact'. At that time the condition we now call autism was called childhood psychosis. The term childhood autism replaced it and is still included in ICD-10 under the general heading 'Pervasive Developmental Disorder', but is not in the latest edition of the DSM. It is apparent that neither, will it be retained in ICD-11, where the term 'Autism Spectrum Disorder' is likely to be used, which is good because we know autism is a lifelong condition and not a condition just of childhood. However, distinguished psychiatrists have continued to use the words 'autism', or 'autistic', in relatively recent papers on psychopathology, in the psychiatric literature, without any reference to autism or autism spectrum disorder (Parnas et al. 2002; Bech 2013).

Distinctions at the phenomenological level

Further confusion may also occur because of the argument, still made by a few psychiatrists, that autism and schizophrenia are one and the same condition. As mentioned in Chapter 3 there is growing genetics research that does not support this view. The literature on schizophrenia increasingly views it also as a developmental disorder, basing this on factors identified in birth cohorts during childhood, differentiating children who later develop schizophrenia from the teen years onwards, from those who do not. Referrals are now often received from early onset psychosis services, and many of the young adults they request advice on do indeed have childhood developmental patterns of shyness and some difficulties in friendship formation, but few if any other suggestions of autism. There are no difficulties with the suggestion that schizophrenia may have different developmental precursors, but there is no evidence that those precursors resemble the specific early child developmental patterns seen in autism.

The distinction between worry, rumination, and mental rigidity

A number of symptoms and behaviours, seen in autism, resemble those seen in other mental disorders (conditions that will be discussed later in this chapter); it is useful to think of these at the symptom level first here. Many examples have been mentioned in previous chapters. These symptoms may mask autism and autism may also mask them. Examples are symptoms of depression and of anxiety.

In Chapter 8, the semi-structured interviewing approach used in the SCAN interview was described, as was the current development of a section on neurodevelopmental disorders. SCAN glossary definitions include guidance on the distinction between symptoms that might be easily confused with each other. In Chapter 3, we touched on the difficulty of differentiating repetitive behaviour due to obsessive compulsive disorder and that due to autism. For example, three relevant symptoms will be covered in the currently developing revision of the SCAN: worry, obsessional rumination, and mental rigidity (the lack of mental flexibility—either in the abnormal adherence to rules, or difficulty experienced with other minor changes) in autism. These are phenomenologically distinct symptoms.[1] Repetitive behaviours could indicate a form of obsessive compulsive disorder or could point to autism. Sometimes the correct diagnosis is reasonably obvious—handwashing rituals are more likely to denote an obsessional condition, lining up objects collected, but otherwise not used for any discernible purpose suggests an autistic phenomenon. As mentioned earlier, the distinction, in less obvious cases, may be gleaned from asking the respondent would they choose to give up this behaviour, if we could give them a medicine that put a stop to it. Patients with OCD can be expected to say yes; those with ASD tend say no. However, both conditions may co-exist, although this is probably rare (Russell et al. 2005).

Symptom masking and amplification

Depression can lead to a high ADOS score (see previous chapter), with the risk that autism will be considered present, when it is not (perhaps more so if the ADOS is carried out by an interviewer not trained and experienced in general psychopathology). This points to the need to distinguish autism like behaviours from the condition itself, the former being more likely to be *secondary to another condition* and the latter, primarily genetically determined, with a clear prior developmental trace to be found in early childhood. Similarly, someone who hardly speaks or looks at their psychiatrist, and has a blank inert face and little non-verbal gesture, may be diagnosed as having depression, who is not depressed, but is autistic. In both cases, amplification and masking of symptoms may lead to the wrong diagnosis, and incorrect advice and treatment may follow, with potentially unwelcome

---

[1] They are described together with distinct rating rules, in the revised SCAN glossary (http://whoscan.org/introduction/).

consequences. Observation over a longer period of time should reveal a different pattern of behaviour, in general, with greater fluctuation in mood and functioning in depression and a striking stability in observed behaviour in autism, although this may be punctuated by very brief moments of deteriorated behaviour, which people with autism often refer to as 'melt downs' (Chapter 4). Such distinctions could be important in evaluating possible risks to self and others.

Just as it must be quite frightening, at first, for an adult who is blind to venture into an unfamiliar part of a city, it is sometimes frightening for a young adult with autism to set foot in a workplace, college, or university for the first time, negotiating unfamiliar people and landmarks and distracting stimuli. They will, quite probably, look anxious and, if asked, may describe symptoms indistinguishable from anxiety; but is this anxiety, for which that diagnosis and the many remarkably effective anxiety treatments is appropriate? There is no evidence that such treatments have a place in these situations.

Under-recognition of autism by psychiatrists has been demonstrated in several studies (Nylander and Gillberg 2001). Rates of autism appear to be greater in inpatients and those who are more severely mentally ill. This is also backed up by a recent study, mentioned in Chapter 2, of random samples of adult patients in contact with mental health services, where only about 1 in 5 cases of autism had come to the attention of their mental health team (approximately 1 in 20 of all cases under their care; Tyrer et al. 2013). Depression and personality disorder were two categories of mental disorder that were found in many of the unrecognized autism cases. The small number of cases of personality disorder tended to attract the designation 'borderline personality disorder'. This might support previous research that ASD can be 'masked' (or misdiagnosed) by such disorders (Rydén et al. 2008).

The contribution of epidemiology to our vigilance and readiness

Epidemiology is helpful to clinical practice because it alerts us to be vigilant about common conditions. How do we know what are common comorbidities of autism? We need to distinguish clinical studies from general population prevalence studies. Studies of the prevalence of comorbidities common in individuals with autism will tell us what to expect if we are seeing comparable populations. However, does that mean that the conditions observed more often are associated?

We know from the results of community prevalence surveys that in adulthood most people with autism are undiagnosed and are not in contact with mental health services (Chapter 1, Epidemiology). Therefore, the small proportion seen in clinical care is unrepresentative of the condition, as it occurs in the general population. It could be that more frequently observed co-occurring conditions represent the processes that lead to referral and recognition. Thus, studies of clinical populations may represent the populations we see clinically, but we cannot infer a particular explanation for such co-occurrences. Community survey data support the long-recognized inference that autism is associated with intellectual disability, with epilepsy and with ADHD. It also points to a concern that suicidal thoughts and actions are more common than expected in autism. However, to date we have not found strong associations between autism and anxiety or depression in our community research. This suggests, perhaps, that adults with autism and anxiety, or depression, are more likely to be referred to specialist clinics. However, there is little if any intrinsic association between these conditions in the way that, for example, epilepsy and intellectual disability are clearly associated with autism, as confirmed in community surveys.

Course and development

Careful consideration of patterns of development and of outcome can be invaluable in differentiating autism from other conditions that we see in adulthood.

For adult psychiatry, a crucial distinction between autism and the mental disorders we commonly see is that the former is developmental and, increasingly, is being diagnosed in early childhood, before or soon after schooling begins. Most of the conditions we see and treat in adults develop from puberty onwards (anxiety may be an exception). Arguably the most valuable method of differentiation is to take a developmental history (Chapter 7). It is not unusual to see an adult who describes a pattern of symptoms and difficulties, particularly socially, suggestive of autism, but on further enquiry, with the help of parents, is not reflected in progress and development in childhood. In psychiatry, we rarely make the effort to contact parents and take a developmental history, a method described in this book in Chapter 7, based on knowledge of normal and atypical development, described in Chapter 3.

A second useful distinction arises from consideration of the course of a clinical presentation, when followed up in the months and years following identification. Developmental disorders tend to follow a stable and quite predictable course, with a small proportion showing some improvement or further deterioration at follow-up (Howlin et al. 2014). Whereas, as we know, the pattern in mental disorders developing after childhood, mood disorders and psychosis, tends more to fluctuation, including relapses, periods of improvement, if not necessarily recovery. Levels of risk to self and others may vary alongside such changes.

In the clinic it is important and useful to ask parents at what age they began to have concerns. When asking about early development, including social development and communication. One should ask them also to think back to a time before these difficulties that are present now, first began to emerge. Symptoms and behaviours associated with autism can worsen in the teen and early adult years (sometimes alongside comorbid depression) so that clarity as to whether symptoms were present in early childhood is important in determining whether autism is the key underlying issue.

A third distinction, not always as useful, but sometimes helpful, is that developmental abnormalities tend to be pervasive. That is they are seen to persist in different contexts. Mental disorders, on the other hand, may at least appear to vary according to context and of course this particularly applies to some forms of anxiety. Positive and negative life events often seem to be associated with corresponding reductions and increases in symptoms with prolonged phases of change. A different pattern seems to apply in autism with shorter phases of response to external factors.[2] Carers, and others who know the patient well, can provide information that casts light on such associations. Patients may be less aware of them.

A fourth, and obvious useful factor to consider, is response (or not) to treatment. This is not entirely straightforward. For example, anxiolytic medication is often found to be somewhat helpful in combating the fears or anxieties described in autism, and clearly can bring relief to the non-autistic anxious adult. Antipsychotic medication may also reduce levels of disturbed behaviour in both (although this is not a recommended treatment in autism). However, in general, patients who are seen in autism clinics, who have had psychiatric treatments, report limited benefit, whereas being diagnosed and supported, with adjustments being made to help them cope, do seem to help the autistic adult, as will be discussed in Part III.

Developmental impairments in social interaction, as mentioned in Chapter 3, are at the heart of what we currently think about autism. However, social functioning can also be strongly affected by any major

---

[2] A striking observation is the rapidity with which a person with autism is able to return to emotional equilibrium, following a disturbing event, in contrast to the prolonged effects of such a disturbing event on other family members.

mental disorder in adulthood and by childhood traumas. It takes time, and the build-up of clinical experience, to differentiate distinctions in the quality of social interaction in autism and in mental disorder. Hopefully, the suggestions made in this section will assist the reader in clarifying, which form of disorder predominates and requires further attention.

Specific comorbidities

Commonly occurring comorbidities are listed in Box 10.1. As mentioned in the earlier part of this chapter, these are co-occurring conditions that you will often see in adult clinical practice, although their associations may simply reflect patterns of referral. Such patterns may change in the future, as services change. Given the lack of consistent information available on these co-occurrences, frequencies, or numbers to expect in given populations will not be suggested. Readers are free to seek out reviews of rates of comorbidity in adulthood within clinical populations. Most of the conditions highlighted by them as being common co-occurrences, are mentioned throughout the remainder of this chapter (i.e. see Box 10.1).

The reader who is unfamiliar with these conditions should refer to published diagnostic criteria (World Health Organization 1993; American Psychiatric Association 2013). Here, we will focus on particular issues that arise during the assessment process that can help with their differentiation.[3]

Autism can be strongly affected by any major mental disorder in adulthood (Chapter 10). It takes time and the build-up of experience to differentiate differences in the quality of social interaction in autism and in mental disorder (e.g. responding to other's expressed feelings).

Disorders of intellectual disability

Mild forms of intellectual disability, in adults who have spoken language, are not always picked up within general psychiatry, and it is likely that this also affects the detection of autism, which is far commoner in this part of the population. Depending on the patient's language development, conventional approaches to psychiatric assessment may be inadequate, in particular, the direct patient interview. Closed questions may generate misleading 'yeah' or 'nay' saying response patterns. Such assessments require more time. The NICE (2012) adult guideline group concluded that any risk assessment of adults with autism should consider the risk of self-harm and of suicide in people with moderate or severe intellectual disabilities (as well as in

---

[3] The use of tests and interviews such as SCAN to identify these conditions is currently being evaluated in local assessment services.

Box 10.1 Commonly seen comorbidities of autism in adulthood

Neurodevelopmental disorders

- Intellectual disability or intellectual disability disorder (IDD).
- Attention deficit hyperactivity disorder (ADHD).
- Social (pragmatic) communication disorder (SCD).
- Communication disorders.
- Developmental coordination disorder (DCD).
- Tick disorder (TD).

Mental disorders in adulthood

- Anxiety.
- Depression.
- Obsessive compulsive disorder.
- Psychosis, schizophrenia.

Other important behaviours and disorders

- Suicidality (thoughts and actions).
- Personality disorder, although sociopathy is rare it is very important to identify this co-occurrence.
- Alcohol abuse.
- Eating disorder.
- Gender dysphoria.

Other conditions

- Epilepsy.
- (The suggestion that dementia is rare in autism is untested).

those with depression). In addition to self-harm, there needs to be alertness to rapid escalation of problems, harm to others, self-neglect, breakdown of family or residential support, and exploitation or abuse by others (NICE, 2012).

Patients seen by different practitioners may be observed to show signs of learning (of which they may be unaware) that certain phrases lead to rewarding responses from the clinician (not being discharged from care, having a preferred medication repeated, or the dose increased). Advice and guidance from a specialist with greater experience with such populations should be considered and may help identify professional learning and development needs.

As just mentioned, autism is much commoner in the presence of intellectual disability. Research on this in adults, both living in care settings and in the community, suggests that it may be commoner than previously thought, and may therefore, go partly undetected (Brugha et al. 2016). In the most profound cases of intellectual disability it may be very difficult to know whether autism is present and this additional knowledge may not alter the care provided.

The observational methods, and the use of accounts by carers described in Chapters 7 and 9, will be particularly valuable in addressing this.

Attention deficit hyperactivity disorder (ADHD)

The knowledge and skills required to assess *ADHD* should be, like those for assessing autism, grounded in the training of adult psychiatrists. Improved proficiency (through additional training), and the use of an apparently cost-effective self-report test questionnaire (Kessler et al. 2005), the ASRS, have helped identify a surprising number of cases in adults, referred for autism assessments, whose ADHD might otherwise go undetected. Most cases seen have either one condition or the other; adult patients with *both* ADHD and autism are seen, but far less often. The implications for treatment are interesting and under researched. ADHD seems to be particularly common in certain subpopulations, such as in adults in custody. ADHD is particularly rewarding to identify, as there is often helpful medical treatment[4] and, of course, the benefits of having official recognition of behaviour that can be viewed as anti-social or asocial.

Social (pragmatic) communication disorder

The term 'Social (Pragmatic) Communication Disorder' is now recommended in DSM-5, in cases in which there are social and pragmatic communication problems similar to those seen in autism, but in the absence of

---

[4] Non- medical advice on coping with adult ADHD is also available from the Royal College of Psychiatrists London: www.rcpsych.ac.uk

repetitive behaviours and sensory differences. A practical and concerning implication is that in some settings, when the autism label is applied, specified forms of care are mandated (or made more accessible), but no such entitlements apply if the questionable distinction is made between autism and 'social communication disorder'. In many years of clinical work the author cannot recall seeing a patient with repetitive behaviours who does not exhibit at least some social and communication difficulties. Quite often patients are seen with social and communication difficulties who do not have rigidity or repetitive behaviours, but who are significantly disabled by the former. Not all research groups accept the requirement in DSM-5 for such behaviours, in making an autism spectrum disorder diagnosis (Waterhouse et al. 2016).

Other forms of Communication Disorders (DSM-5), although rarely seen in the context of adult autism clinics, may present in a subtle form if overlooked by the referrer, as these neurodevelopmental disorders normally present in early childhood and are therefore, unlikely to be overlooked throughout childhood into adulthood. A speech and language assessment should be considered, and neuropsychologists with a particular interest in this area may also be very helpful.

Developmental coordination disorder

Gross and fine motor skills are particularly important in general development and are often delayed in adults with autism and occur also independently of autism. Neurologists seem to pay more attention to them than do child psychiatrists (Gillberg and Kadesjo 2003). The term Developmental Coordination Disorder (DCD) is now officially recognized as a condition in its own right (American Psychiatric Association 2013). DCD can also occur in association with ADHD.

Anxiety

Anxiety appears to be ubiquitous in clinical populations in which autism occurs. Patients with autism often have difficulties in describing emotions (alexithymia). Patients with autism can describe what they do, or are thinking, but have difficulty in describing how they are feeling. With specific prompting, they may be able, to describe autonomic symptoms of anxiety and, again with difficulty, experiencing these feelings more so in specific settings. As with depression, where the same problem applies, the clinician needs to think carefully what to say to or ask the patient, to avoid misunderstanding. Of course, what the patient says in reply might reflect very different issues, such as over sensitivity to topics that trigger anxiety or irritation.

Social phobia (social anxiety disorder) is a common presentation in adults referred for an assessment for possible autism, particularly, as social phobia includes acute self-awareness and a fear of not appearing normal. Some time should be given to considering social phobia before proceeding with a detailed autism assessment.

Depression

It is remarkable how difficult it can be for the autistic adult to describe what it feels like to be depressed. Far more time needs to be given to such assessments. Clearly, as stated earlier, non-verbal signs suggestive of depression simply cannot be relied upon as a guide. Vegetative signs of depression (so called biological symptoms) will be less difficult for the patient to describe including increased lethargy, loss of interest, appetite, and weight, and also sleep disturbance. Questions about time course may be difficult, as the concept of time may be poorly developed. Self-identity and the concept of self,[5] may also complicate understanding and helping such patients. There needs to be, and has not been, a thorough and systematic evaluation of methods for assessing depression in adults with autism. This has yet to be carried out with the revised SCAN interview, assessing and cross questioning, simultaneously, both forms of psychopathology.

Lack of interest in peers should particularly be enquired about from early childhood, if autism is suspected in a depressed adult. As stated previously, lack of interest in interacting with peers is clearly described in depression in adulthood, and accounts based solely on observation of adulthood are potentially misleading. However, a tendency to choose to interact with someone much older or younger, may persist into adulthood in autism and this is something an adult observer can note, without having known the patient as a child.

Obsessive compulsive disorder

This has been discussed in detail earlier in this book, including earlier in this chapter. There is no substitute for clinical experience with both conditions. As mentioned before, OCD may be missed by practitioners who mainly see autism, and autism may be missed or incorrectly attributed by practitioners who have not had guided experience in assessing autism.

---

[5] Difficulties with sexual identity appear to be increasingly reported by adult autism clinics, but we do not know if this is part of a pattern of reporting to all adult and child psychiatric services.

Psychosis

There has been a high level of concern in some autism support networks and communities that psychosis is often incorrectly diagnosed in adults on the autism spectrum. This can occur, but only occasionally and when it does, brief reactive psychosis should be considered before schizophrenia thus keeping open the possibility of remission without the need for a prolonged period of treatment that is not necessary. Psychosis is, perhaps, more likely to occur in very damaged individuals in long-term dependency and care settings, where some of the odd repetitive behaviours, listed in Chapter 9, will be helpful in differentiating psychosis and autism. Beginning with the Chapter 2, on developing awareness of autism, one would hope that psychiatrists learning about autism will now be open to considering this as a possibility, in their long-term care patient populations. Meticulous attention to the assessment of both conditions is the best way to address this and particularly in evaluating symptoms at interview.[6] Factors that may help identify schizophrenia include its later onset, a period of gradual deterioration before positive psychotic symptoms emerge, and a lack of the non-verbal communication abnormalities characteristic of autism.

When discussing treatment, and particularly the use of medication in Part III, we will discuss the high level of sensitivity and elevated risk of side effects to psychotropic medication seen in this population. Persistent side effects, even when antipsychotic medication doses have been reduced, should also be an alerting signal to the possibility of a neurodevelopmental disorder and, perhaps, particularly autism. See also Case Study B in Chapter 2.

Suicidality (thoughts and actions)

A growing number of studies point to the likelihood that risk of suicide is increased in the adult autism population. Our as yet unpublished general population data, also gives some support to this.[7] Psychiatrists working in acute and trauma settings, and with older isolated male populations, should be particularly vigilant to this. The fact that many patients (speaking of those who survive suicide attempts) are living socially isolated lives, it is very important to think autism before discharging such patients, in effect, to a life often without care and support.

---

[6] The SCAN approach, under development, may well be the way forward.

[7] Jordanova, V. (2012). Suicidality in adults with Autistic Spectrum Disorders. Preliminary findings presented to the World Psychiatric Association Section on Epidemiology and Public Health 2012, Sau Paulo, Brazil.

Personality disorder

The description of schizoid personality disorder in ICD-10 could be viewed as bearing a remarkable similarity to a form of autism (or of 'Asperger syndrome'). Adult autism clinics are probably often asked to see patients who, in the past, might have been labelled as schizoid. One need only compare the quantity of scientific research, published annually on these two categories, to realize which has the firmer base in our scientific efforts.

ICD-10 includes the idea that personality disorder can be considered a form of developmental disorder. This has often been found to be a useful way of viewing this concept.

As psychiatrists refer more and more patients to adult autism clinics, we see more cases where they have used personality disorder labels, including 'borderline', 'emotionally unstable', 'inadequate'. Experience of seeing adults with the borderline label is that they are usually unrecognized cases of autism in women, who have great difficulties with social and emotional functioning. They may have experienced more abuse due to their vulnerabilities, lack of communication skills, and social understanding. Placed with peers who self-harm (or with eating disorders) they may imitate such behaviours. Nevertheless, sometimes the borderline label is the more convincing of the two. Colleagues working with complex, challenging adults, in inpatient care, are more likely to see patients with both kinds of psychopathology.

Sociopathy comorbid with autism is occasionally seen. We have no idea how rare this is. Cases have been referred more often by the courts and the criminal justice system, than by NHS colleagues, and can be some of the most challenging and concerning cases we are ever asked to advise on. This will clearly have a bearing on advice to the courts (Part III).

Epilepsy

The statistically significant association with epilepsy has been mentioned earlier. Epilepsy should be routinely enquired into, in autism. It is particularly common when intellectual disability is also present and is a major part of the work of intellectual disability psychiatry in childhood and adulthood.

Conclusion

Once a diagnosis has been clearly made on the autism spectrum, including disentangling psychiatric comorbidities, further specific investigations may be needed in order to advise and develop a care plan. This applies particularly to more severely affected individuals, which explains why the necessary resources and facilities are more likely to be available to intellectual disability services. There is much more limited experience of the benefits and indications for additional assessments, in the more able adult population with autism, as shall be seen in Chapter 11, which concludes Part II of this book.

Chapter 11

Detailed needs assessment

Introduction

In previous chapters, in Part II, we looked at how to decide on whether autism should be considered and, if so, the various approaches to deciding on whether it should be diagnosed. This chapter pre-supposes that we have a patient, who we have decided is significantly affected on the autism spectrum, and who needs closer attention, for example because informal support in family and educational settings has not been sufficient to address concerns. It also presupposes the existence of a service, if not necessarily designated as specialist, which is, at least, sufficiently resourced to be able to offer a more detailed profile of needs, with a view to developing a management plan.

We focus now on those further assessments that may be *needed*. By need we do not mean 'wished for' or 'demanded' but, rather, we mean 'potentially beneficial to this patient' (in a specifiable sense). Thus, any further assessment should only be carried out if it is likely to add information that will help (and not hinder) the patient in the future.

The first part of this chapter re-iterates briefly the importance of a detailed profiling of the way in which autism affects the person—all cases being unique. The second part considers 'status' and 'outcome' measures, which have been used in clinical trials in autism, in adults, which both add to the patient profile, and which may be a baseline on which to evaluate future progress. The third part looks at the input that different disciplines can bring—multi-disciplinary assessment approaches, being widely endorsed in child and increasingly adult services, for people with autism. Finally, briefly, mention will be made of other tests that are largely still in the research laboratory, as their value in individual case work has not been established, but which could be helpful in particular cases.

Detailed individual profile of autism phenotype

Chapter 12 will begin with discussing with the patient the results of his or her assessment findings, because that is a key part of discussing care and management. One of the first things patients often ask is whether their condition is called autism, or Asperger syndrome?[1] Do we need to consider this in an assessment? Under DSM-IV (and at the time of writing the still current ICD-10) there is the option to specify subtypes of 'Pervasive Developmental Disorder', including Asperger's disorder, childhood autism, etc. With the publication of DSM-5 the list of subtypes has been dropped. Instead the diagnostician is encouraged to use the umbrella term, Autism Spectrum Disorder (ASD), only. It is for the clinician to explain this sensitively (given prior expectations of the patient and any family). It is expected that ICD-11 will follow a similar pathway and replace the term Pervasive Developmental Disorder, with the umbrella term Autism Spectrum Disorder.

Under DSM-5 the clinician is then encouraged to code the severity of ASD in terms of level of support needed. Several specifiers may then be added, the most important being presence of intellectual disability. In this chapter we will discuss further assessment of cognitive ability. Another key term, often used (interchangeably), is 'adaptive ability', which is always going to be important, and which is a key predictor of outcome in follow-up cohort research (Howlin et al. 2014). Other specifiers, which it is recommended to include (under DSM-5), would be the presence of comorbidities, such as ADHD, if also present. Any significant physical ill-health would of course be added here. A summary discharge letter to primary care should list these key findings succinctly (and the name of any key actions recommended).

The advanced diagnostic assessment

For a more advanced diagnostic workup, if full semi-structured interview assessments have not yet been undertaken, *and* if we are dealing with an adult who is significantly impaired who will need regular or continuing help and support, the case can be made for conducting detailed and full assessments of lifelong development and of current behaviour. The suggested instruments are already described in previous chapters, in Part II. The developmental history should be documented, if possible from early childhood, using the DISCO (Leekam et al. 2002; Wing 1993, 2000; Wing et al. 2002) or the ADI-R (Lord et al. 1994), or other approaches listed in Chapter 7. Current behaviour should be assessed with the ADOS (Lord et al. 1994).

If it is felt that a follow-up 'outcome' assessment is envisaged, following a period of intervention, the evolving literature on the use of the ADOS as a

---

[1] An issue first raised in the Preface, again in Chapter 1 and also in some later chapters.

measure of change should be consulted. Work on lower ability children is being undertaken (Gotham et al. 2009, 2012).

However, in primary care, such additional detailed assessments are rarely feasible. Indeed, the necessity for them should be questioned if the person is functioning reasonably well throughout most of their life with some informal support, apart from occasional crises during which additional crisis support may be needed briefly. The rationale for this will be considered further in Part III.

Status and outcome measures used in clinical trials in adulthood

A measure of health or of functional status can be considered to be a status measure, at any time it is used (as in the 'present state'), or it can be used as an outcome measure, where it is possible to use it to infer a response to some specified intervention. With Professor Pat Howlin, the author's research group recently reviewed the literature on outcome measures for use in clinical trials in adult autism (Brugha et al. 2015). The measures that have been used more than occasionally may also have some use in clinical settings in which a more detailed assessment is needed. Most commonly used were the Clinical Global Impression (CGI) rating scale and the Yale–Brown Obsessive Compulsive Scale (YBOCS). Other measures used occasionally will also be mentioned here.

We searched for clinical trials in adults with autism spectrum disorders. Searches were limited to articles in English published between 1960 and January 2013. We found 29 intervention studies that we included in our review; most were based on small samples and often lacked any comparison groups. Thirteen treatment trials (all but four pharmacological) involved randomized control studies. None of the studies reviewed, specifically, assessed the sensitivity, reliability, validity, or even general utility of the measures they used for adults with ASD. The only publication identified that discusses these issues in detail was a review paper, on child pharmacological intervention studies, by Arnold and colleagues (2000), using a consensus based approach, we would like to see adopted for research on adults. We divided the reviewed measures into those that covered partially or completely, core components of autism and other measures, which considered factors that might be affected or important in this population (Box 11.1).

The Ritvo–Freeman Real-life Rating Scale (RF–RLRS; Freeman et al. 1986), was the most frequently used global measure of ASD symptoms, albeit, only in pharmacological interventions, which was developed for use in children. It is an observational measure of symptoms of autism. It

> **Box 11.1 Selective status and outcome measures used in intervention evaluations in adolescents and in adults**
>
> **Global measures**
>
> - Ritvo-Freeman Real-life Rating Scale (RF-RLRS; Freeman et al. 1986).
> - Autism Behavior Checklist (ABC; Krug et al. 1980).
> - Social Responsiveness scale (SRS; Constantino and Gruber 2002).
>
> **Specific domains**
>
> Yale–Brown Obsessive Compulsive Scale (Y-BOCS [full or modified forms]; (Goodman et al. 1989a,b).
>
> **Non-autism specific measures**
>
> - Clinical Global Impression rating scale (CGI; Guy 1976).
> - Aberrant Behavior Checklist (ABC; Aman et al. 1985).
> - Maladaptive Sub-scale of the Vineland Adaptive Behavior Scales (VABS; Sparrow et al. 1984).
>
> **Change in cognitive ability.**
>
> - Assessment of working memory (Bodner et al. 2012).
> - Assessment of executive function (Garcia-Villamisar and Hughes 2007).
>
> Adapted from *International Journal of Methods in Psychiatric Research*, 24, Brugha, T. S., Doos, L., Tempier, A., Einfeld, S., & Howlin, P, Outcome measures in intervention trials for adults with autism spectrum disorders; a systematic review of assessments of core autism features and associated emotional and behavioural problems, pp. 99–115, Copyright 2015, with permission from John Wiley and Sons.

includes sensory motor behaviours (Subscale I: hand-flapping, rocking, pacing, etc.), social relationships (Subscale II: appropriate responses to interaction attempts, initiating appropriate physical interactions), affectual reactions (Subscale III: abrupt changes in affect, crying, temper outbursts), sensory responses (Subscale IV: agitated by noises, rubbing surfaces, sniffing self or objects), and language (Subscale V: communicative use of language, initiating appropriate verbal communication). The items reflect behaviours commonly observed in adults with ASD, across the ability range, and are scored on a 4-point scale: (0 = never; 3 = almost always). An overall score is derived from the mean value of each of the 5 subscale scores, (range for overall score, 0.42–2.58). As an observational scale, the RF-RLRS can only be used to evaluate change in study participants who are repeatedly observed by trained raters. However, Arnold and colleagues (Arnold et al. 2000) also found poor reliability between different sites. The review describes the use of other less often used measures of symptoms of autism (Brugha et al. 2015), including the Autism Behavior Checklist (ABC; Krug et al. 1980), the Social Responsiveness scale (SRS; Constantino and Gruber 2002). The measures listed in the previous paragraph, including the ADOS, had not been used as measures of change in the trials we found.

In regard to measures of specific autism domains, there was no consistent use of standardized measures designed specifically to assess social competence in autism (Brugha et al. 2015). In order to measure repetitive behaviours, the Yale–Brown Obsessive Compulsive Scale was used in six studies (Y-BOCS [full or modified forms]; Goodman et al. 1989a,b). The reader is cautioned to examine the items in this scale carefully before deciding whether they are appropriate in a particular population or case. As was pointed out earlier, repetitive behaviours in autism and in obsessive compulsive disorder are not the same phenomenologically, although that distinction may be difficult to determine sometimes, unless the patient is able to describe, verbally, how they perceive and view their repetitive behaviours.

Non-autism specific measures were, used the most, these being the Clinical Global Impression rating scale (CGI; Guy 1976), which was used in 9 autism intervention trials. The CGI is very familiar to psychiatrists because of its use in RCTs of severe mental illness, so it will not be described here, other than to say that it is based on ratings of symptom severity and improvement, using seven-point scales, rated by a clinician who is also assessing the patient clinically. The Aberrant Behavior Checklist (ABC; Aman et al. 1985) was used in trials on severely intellectually disabled individuals. The Maladaptive Sub-scale of the Vineland Adaptive Behavior Scales (VABS; Sparrow et al. 1984) was used in three trials, but there is uncertainty regarding its sensitivity to change).

Other areas covered included aggression and self-injury, mood states, self-esteem, and quality of life (Brugha et al. 2015). Two studies assessed change in cognitive ability. Bodner and colleagues (2012) reported improvements in working memory, following a trial of propranolol. Executive function improvement was shown in a supported employment trial of Garcia-Villamisar and Hughes (2007).

One further study (Narayanan 2010), used magnetic resonance imaging to assess response to propranolol, which reported some improvement in brain connectivity.

The European Union Medicines Agency has prepared draft guidance on the development and clinical evaluation of treatments for autism, which also covers the topic of outcome measures and the issue of harm and its avoidance (http://www.ema.europa.eu/docs/en_GB/document_library/Scientific_guideline/2016/03/WC500202650.pdf).

Input to assessment that different disciplines can bring—multi-disciplinary approaches

According to the adult autism care pathway for Leicester and Leicestershire a holistic assessment of need 'should be undertaken by the appropriate members of the Health and Social Care Teams, who have experience in working with people with autism. This will include Social Workers, Psychologists, Community Mental Health Nurses, Occupational Therapists, and Psychiatrists. The pathway follows steps similar to those graphically displayed at the beginning of Part II:

> 'The professional(s) undertaking this process should be those best suited to the individual's main areas of need. For example, if mental health difficulties are part of the picture, then a Community Nurse / Psychiatrist / Psychologist would be best placed to lead a needs assessment; while if the needs are primarily in the social care field, then a Social Worker should lead.
>
> The assessment of need may highlight certain areas requiring specialist intervention and support, for example risk behaviours/offending. Referrals should be made to the appropriate organizations for these to be further assessed and managed, for example the Probation Service and/or Forensic Mental Health services.
>
> Each professional group will have its own assessment tools and measures for assessing need and monitoring progress. For the purposes of the Pathway, two key outcome-based measures are being recommended for general use (see below). It is important to incorporate outcome measures at this stage of the assessment, to ensure that the focus of any intervention chosen is clear, and to help monitor progress'.[2]

In addition to psychiatry, several disciplines may have particular insights to offer, psychology including neuropsychology, speech and language therapy, social work, occupational therapy. A further strength that comes from having several different disciplines involved, who may be able to view the

---

[2] http://www.leicspart.nhs.uk/Library/v2AdultPathwayWeb240215.pdf.

patient in different environments and different contexts, is that the significance of initial concerns about risks, to self or others, can be explored more thoroughly and discussed at team meetings. Furthermore, the patient may communicate more willingly with one member of the team, who may thus be able to develop a shared approach to minimizing risk that the patient is prepared to accept co-operatively. In developing an approach to risk assessment and management, the NICE (2012) adult clinical guideline development group pointed to the importance of being 'aware of the sensitivity of some people with autism to changes in their physical or social environment and the possibility of the very rapid escalation of problems including risk-related problems due to changes in the social or physical environment'.

Psychology

Several branches of psychology can contribute to a further assessment and clearer pointers to subsequent care planning including educational, clinical, occupational, and neuropsychology.

Cognitive and academic ability will be an important determinant of the sorts of work and employment settings in which the individual is able to function. Problems in *processing speed* may hold up a student's academic progress, but such students can be helped, for example, by being given extra time in examinations. It will also help with choices of the kinds of support (s)he may need in accommodation. Without such tests, one is relying on descriptions from carers, who can sometimes under estimate how well the person can manage with independence. Problems with processing speed, in further education and university settings, may pose particular difficulties in keeping up with lectures, completion of written course work by deadlines set by tutors. Provision of a note taker (and extra time in exams) are all considered reasonable adjustments, within the education system in Great Britain, where local education authorities have responsibilities for funding additional supports (see Chapter 13).

As mentioned in Chapter 3, executive functioning deficits can affect organizational ability, time keeping, planning and prioritizing, and multi-tasking, all of which will be important as the person moves into living independently, studying at higher education level, and in many employment tasks. As will be discussed in Chapter 13, there are a number of steps that can be taken to support the person with these difficulties.

Inattention and distractibility will also be potential stumbling blocks, at college and in some employment settings. The possibility of ADHD should be considered, although psychometric testing may not be all that helpful in evaluating the severity of ADHD symptoms, which should also be assessed, clinically.

Speech and language therapy

If the adult has well developed speech since childhood, the assessment should look into speech pragmatics (understanding and using language for social purposes) and the ability to use language to narrate, in an organized way. In adults with limited language ability, the speech and language assessment should consider the patient's functioning in expressive and receptive language (these are covered in the developmental assessments, DISCO and PPBS, described in Chapter 7). Particularly valuable insights may also come from a combined approach to assessment of communication by a speech and language therapist and a psychologist working together. The speech and language therapist can also be useful in convincing carers of the language abilities of patients—when carers overestimate a person's understanding. Given that disturbed behaviours can be due to frustrations in communication they can often help greatly in this area, particularly with the minimization of potential escalations in risk behaviour.

Speech and language therapists will also make use of the kinds of assessments that have been described in this and earlier chapters in Part II. Given their interest in language and communication, and speech pragmatics, they may be the first to raise the possibility that a case of autism has been overlooked. Depending on the structure and culture of the medical hierarchy, with which they work, the approach they take to alerting such issues may vary, and the good psychiatrist will take an interest in the finer points of their assessments, in those few cases in which such assessments are provided. With the older adult, speech and language therapists will also be alert to signs of cognitive decline.

In Chapter 9, we discussed the assessment of some of the qualities of speech that the Speech and Language Therapist will be in a position to study more systematically. This included gauging the level of non-verbal comprehension as well as specific examples of communication difficulty, tone of voice, and a voice that is too quiet or loud. Observing these signs may well be a trigger to action, and possibly to a referral, if available for a speech and language therapy assessment.

Social work

The term social work has very different meanings in different cultures and societies. With the development of Community Care, social workers in Great Britain lost much of their front line role in directing and supporting clients (the term preferred to the word 'patient'). Instead, they were given a brokerage role, focusing on assessment of care needs (often termed social care needs); they also had, and have, access to community care funds to meet needs. Assessment has tended to be influenced very much by this brokerage and prioritization process. In very recent years with the severe cut backs in social care funding, assessment of eligibility to access community care funding has meant that only those, either in crisis or at impending risk of crisis, are deemed to be supportable with community care resources. In Great Britain social workers are mainly employed and funded by local government, but many health care providers either do, or did employ them (hospitals, community health and mental health services, large charitable service providers). Chapter 14 will be devoted to considering social care in more detail.

Areas particularly relevant to the assessment role of social workers cover all of the domains already considered in Part II of this book. Therefore social workers will be expected to have an understanding of all aspects of disability, physical and mental and to case manage. One's experience has been that they were the most alert profession at recognizing the existence, in society, of adults on the autism spectrum and their care needs and, in view of this, they were the first to put in place training for their profession. One will often recommend, in a discharge letter from the assessment clinic to the primary care (GP) service, from which the patient was first referred, that in case of future crises, social care services should be considered first (rather than mental health services, assuming that there are no significant mental health issues). This applies particularly if there are concerns about the vulnerability of the patient and the need to consider safeguarding issues, requiring a more detailed assessment of risks.

Social workers clearly need to be aware of and able to understand information on cognitive functioning. A classic error that may occur, without sufficient training and experience, is taking literally claims of independence capabilities of an adult on the spectrum who is lacking in insight or awareness of how certain responses to questions can be misinterpreted (and failing to speak to carers). They also need to be able to evaluate adaptive functioning and socialization, both of which should be well documented, assuming the assessment guidance here and in previous chapters has been followed. These topics will also be returned to in Chapter 14.

Occupational therapy

Clearly occupational therapists will have a key role in assessing independent living skills and what training in such skills is needed. Occupational therapists are often part of general adult mental health teams (unlike many of the other specialities listed in this chapter). Therefore, they too, have a potentially important role in alerting us to the possibility of under recognized autism. Further discussion of their role will be included in Chapter 14, on care in the community.

Occupational therapists, as a profession, have taken a particular interest in looking at sensory differences (Chapters 7 and 8), and suggesting ways of supporting patients who have difficulties in these areas. With very disabled individuals on the spectrum, any action that seems to improve quality of life and, perhaps, ease burden on carers, is worthy of consideration particularly if it helps overcome social isolation. Hopefully clinical trials evaluating such approaches will emerge in due course.

Quality of life

Perhaps the topic of quality of life (QOL) should have been one of the first to be covered, on assessment, rather than one of the last. Several years ago, extending the adult epidemiological research to the adult intellectual disability population, no measures appropriate to the topic of autism in adulthood could be identified. Perkins has largely confirmed this in a useful overview chapter on quality of life (Perkins 2016), in Scott Wright's collection of papers on autism spectrum disorder in mid and later life (Wright 2016).

Five domains are generally considered to be of importance to quality of life, physical well-being, material well-being, social well-being, development and activity, emotional well-being. There are widely used measures of QOL, including those used in health economic evaluations, in randomized controlled trials (RCTs) of clinical effectiveness. When the topic comes up in the context of research into the epidemiology of mental disorders (and autism), the range of measures used tends to cover all of these domains, albeit with less scope for harmonization with QOL measures used elsewhere, thus limiting comparison. Of these domains, physical well-being and physical health may be particularly neglected.

Given the limited options for 'treatment' in relation to autism in adulthood, QOL is a particularly important consideration in assessment and, of course, in developing a care plan in which there is personal choice. Although not easy to unpick in individuals from this population, QOL will be one of the best options for being helpful. We will return to the topic of QOL in Part III.

Other tests

In cases where there are other concerns about brain development and functioning, a range of imaging and electrophysiological investigations may sometimes be considered. A cautious approach to such options is to consider the possible benefits of any additional tests with colleagues, with clinical expertise in these areas, before subjecting patients to tests that may be distressing for them. New options for progress may emerge in the future.

Part III

Care and Intervention after Diagnosis

Having covered a range of approaches to diagnostic assessment and to further assessment of need in Part II, in Part III, we will look at options for care and intervention for those who are clearly significantly affected on the autism spectrum. In Chapter 12, we will look at options for treatment, in the way we understand that term in medicine and psychiatry. In Chapter 13, we will begin by acknowledging that autism is a disability (or, as some with the condition prefer it, a set of differences in ability), for which adjustments can be made that improve the lives of patients and, indeed, their carers, in terms of sharing of responsibilities and burden. We will return to principles of social care, raised briefly, in the present chapter. This topic will be further extended in Chapter 14, which looks at the role of wider society, including policy as it affects other areas of life, such as employment, education, housing, access to leisure and other community amenities. Finally, in Chapter 15, we will reflect, briefly, on what difference this learning has made to our professional role in psychiatry, to speculate on what changes the future may bring, and to talk about how we continue to develop our knowledge and skills and research into the future.

Chapter 12

Approaches to treatment and care

Limitations on what is known and what can be done

This chapter commences on a stark negative note. Strictly speaking, there are no evidence based (trial proven) treatments for autism in adulthood. That does not mean that there is nothing we can do. Part III of this book will hopefully make that clear. One could ask what would an evidence-based treatment for adult autism be, if it existed? Able and articulate adults, with the condition, should be listened to in relation to this question. As some of them view it, autism is a different way of being. It is being a particular kind of person. They have said they see no reason for changing the way they are. What they want is help with the negative consequences of autism, including poor mental health, economic and social exclusion. This 'difference' viewpoint is set out and argued in the *Lancet* editorial (2016), 'Pride in autistic diversity', which draws attention to the strengths and unusual abilities and skills that can come with being autistic.

As the *Lancet* article points out, there are persons who are much more severely affected with autism, for whom such a perspective brings limited consolation. For them day to day life is a struggle and the only solution, often seems to be to withdraw totally from life and the world outside, where they live (or even into their bedroom). Subsequent correspondence published by the Lancet also emphasized that point.

Introducing the patient to their assessment outcome and options for moving forward

The first step in intervention is to give to the patient the results of their assessment, and the second is to look at where one can find reliable evidence on care, if that is wanted and needed. As was mentioned earlier, with the consent of the patient, it is sensible for carers who have been involved in the assessment to be present at such a key discussion.

Naming conventions used in discussions with patients and carers

For many years, the author has recommended using the combined terms 'autism' and 'Asperger syndrome', when giving the results of the assessment to the patient (and if agreed to their carers). This has helped to avoid a couple of the legacy problems discussed in earlier chapters, although it may have limited 'future proof' value. First, the removal of the term 'Asperger' from the latest recommendations in classification, avoids the concern that some patients given that label may have, that they have lost their diagnosis. Yes, this is a very literal interpretation of what has happened, but it is a real concern for those who view it that way. Second, both terms have their value. As pointed out in the Preface, some health care systems, including our own in Great Britain, planners and commissioners regard the term autism as meaning people with intellectual disability, who are also autistic. For them the term 'Asperger syndrome' refers to able individuals with autistic traits. Before we dismiss that dichotomy, we need to point out that it highlights the fact that both groups need services.

The title of this book, using both terms, was designed as a 'hook' to bring it to the attention of readers alerted by either of these meanings. The potential for misunderstanding due to these two names being thought of as exclusive is probably gradually disappearing. A new name could replace them in the future if, hoped for, growth in understanding of its biology emerges, eventually bringing valid biomarkers. Third, saying that the patient should feel free to use the term of their choice, depending on who they are talking to, gives them a choice (which may be more comfortable). With their peers, they may prefer words such as 'Asperger' or '*aspie*', a colloquial term. When seeking health and social care resources and support, they might be advised that it is more prudent to use the medical term *autism*.

Treatment goals and targets

Any discussion about intervention, or treatment, should include a consideration of the targets of treatment, the role of patients (and the public) in choosing what their wishes and objectives are. Can a goal be measured? How long might it take to achieve? What would you change if you could change it?

Patients rarely mention an element of their own condition that they want to change. On the contrary, there is probably a strong leaning towards sameness, not change. Reduction in suffering due to symptoms of anxiety, and other kinds of distress, and help with the consequences of their condition, are most often mentioned (and often have been partly addressed before they realize they might need an autism assessment). Families may, of course, point to risk behaviours including self-harm and challenging behaviour. They will also point to neglect of self-care, personal appearance, problems in facing challenges such as social interaction, employment, keeping in touch with friends. These potential differences in goals, preferences, and wishes require reconciling. Always the patient's preferences must take first place. Making choices calls on skills that may be lacking in autism, including planning and considering the future, making use of limited executive functioning ability. Support in making choices, therefore, may be very important. None of us like to be told to give up an activity or behaviour we enjoy, even though risk may be attached to it (for example, high risk sporting pursuits); establishing the sort of collaboration that may be most effectives in minimizing risk will be all the more difficult unless vulnerabilities in social communication are recognized and adjusted to, as part of a risk management plan.

Acceptance and options for care and adjustment where treatment cannot be offered

Given that there are no immediate obvious treatment options, it is crucial to point out that much can be achieved through accepting and learning about what it means to be on the autism spectrum. We will develop this in the next two chapters on social care and societal adjustment. The importance to the patient and family of thinking about learning to live with autism, cannot be overestimated. An initial step, particularly for example for a patient in employment, will be to decide who to share the diagnosis with.

It is not usually the case that adult patients ask about the advisability of treatments that they have heard about. They usually recognize that making adjustments and having support are the way forward. This seems to contrast strikingly with the considerable energy and effort that some parents put into trying to find a treatment for an autistic child while it is still growing and rapidly developing. Advice on where to turn to for evidence is crucial.

Guidelines and sources of evidence on clinical effectiveness

Fortunately there is help available in identifying what to consider, in terms of intervention and treatment, from national, government supported reviews.

The most influential of these, already referred to often in this book, was produced, for the National Health Service (NHS) in England and Wales, by NICE[1] (National Institute for Health and Clinical Excellence (Great Britain) 2012).[2] Medical and psychosocial interventions were systematically reviewed. Studies found were of generally poor quality. Five studies of medical interventions were of fair quality. Positive findings on education (e.g. vocabulary), and social and adaptive skills, were of short-term duration. Antipsychotic medication was associated with improvements in challenging behaviours. The guidance recommended that medication should only be considered for challenging behaviour when psychological and social approaches have been unsuccessful and there are concerns about risk.

The NICE systematic review (2012) and guidance was reviewed in 2016. However, because there was no new significant evidence, that would lead clearly to practice change, NICE deferred further reviewing of the evidence. There is a provision in the procedures followed by NICE, that if there is a major new finding of substantive clinical importance, it will issue a note to that effect. The reader may check the current up to date position, when reading this.

A second, publicly funded, systematic review and guideline, has been produced in the USA (Lounds Taylor et al. 2012) applicable to adolescents and young adults on the autism spectrum. The conclusion was that few studies have been conducted on treatment approaches for this age group. There was little evidence on specific treatment approaches. Most of the available studies were of poor quality. Studies of educational and adaptive functioning were short-term and suggested some limited effects on social skills and on functioning. There were a small number of medication studies of fair quality, but the only evidence to come was of limited effectiveness in the treatment of challenging behaviours.

A second approach to checking for evidence is a rolling programme of evidence reviews, carried out in the UK by Research Autism (http://researchautism.net/). Most of the interventions reviewed are on children, but any relevant adult studies are also evaluated and categorized as such, according to age range covered. This website resource has a further value in that it lists all claims for interventions. Therefore anyone who hears about a particular 'therapy' and searchers for it, has a good chance of finding a

---

[1] Since renamed the National Institute for Health and Care Excellence, to take account of evidence on (social) care.

[2] Scotland has similar guidance in the form of SIGN documents. A growing number of countries have developed similar evidence review and guidance for their own services contexts, for example the US Agency for Healthcare Research and Quality.

description of it here, and sources of information. The site is fearless in pointing to lack of evidence of effectiveness, to unfounded claims and also, flags up concerns about potential harm that could arise. Criteria for rating the quality of research evidence are applied consistently. The resource is backed up by a panel of experts.[3] Since January 2017 Research Autism has functioned under the longstanding umbrella of the UK National Autistic Society. A summary of the evidence is published in book form every five years and is on my recommended reading list (Flemming et al. 2016).

A separate systematic review of outcome measures, used in clinical trials (Brugha et al. 2015) was referred to in Chapter 11.[4] Although not designed primarily to look at intervention evidence, the findings were broadly similar to those summarized in the above reviews. Importantly, for further evidence development, it was concluded that a major obstacle is the paucity of evidence on the validity, and sensitivity to change, of the outcome measures being used in treatment trials in adults.

What works?

Given the above findings from independent systematic reviews, we will focus here on three areas where there seems to be some evidence of benefit from specified interventions, albeit from studies of limited quality. The key issue is what is effective in the longer-term, and not just in the short-term, particularly in relation to psychosocial interventions.

Pharmacotherapy

An important point is that pharmacotherapies do not necessarily have the same effects in children as in adults (Doyle et al. 2014). Therefore, evidence from studies in adults will only be considered further.

Claims for the value of antidepressants, as helping in interfering repetitive behaviours, are not endorsed by independent reviewers.[5]

For the control of challenging behaviours and irritability, antipsychotics do appear to have a role that is more widely endorsed in independent

---

[3] The author is a member of the advisory panel.

[4] Professor Pat Howlin, co-author of this systematic review of outcome measures, also advised on the two national systematic reviews cited here.

[5] A review by Research Autism (http://researchautism.net/) of the place of antidepressants in autism (in any age group), was updated and due to be posted online in early 2017, which concluded that there was no evidence that they have a place in the treatment of autism.

reviews. However, the NICE review (2012) advises that all non-medical approaches must have been attempted first, to address the behavioural problems: 'in addition to the potential to manage behaviour and reduce harm, it has been suggested that pharmacological interventions may also improve response rates to psychological interventions that are aimed at core autism symptoms (Findling, 2005; Malone et al., 2005; McDougle et al., 2003), and may assist individuals with autism to live outside of institutional settings (Posey & McDougle, 2001)'.

It is recognized that pharmacotherapeutic approaches appear to carry an increased likelihood of adverse side effects in this population. Caution in their use is recommended in this population. Nevertheless, these drugs are widely used particularly for children and adults with autism and intellectual disability. However, anything further on that observation would be beyond the scope of this book on adults of average or higher functioning.

Adaptive skills

Behavioural analysis and reinforcement methods, developed in children, have been subject to limited evaluation in adolescents and some promise is claimed (Turygin and Matson 2014). Systematic reviews, quoted earlier, have also reported limited short-term benefits in adaptive functioning, but longer-term outcome evaluations will be needed to determine whether these can be viewed as effective treatments, rather than support interventions, for example, during transitions into independent living.

Psychosocial and community interventions

A review of psychosocial interventions for adults with autism found that there were very few studies of adequate quality, and those that there were used social cognition training, or Applied Behaviour Analysis (ABA; Bishop-Fitzpatrick et al. 2013). The lead author's review of psychosocial, and community-based interventions for adults discussed the topic of ABA, which is regarded as the key evidence-based approach to reducing behaviours that interfere with functioning in social settings, in children. ABA has been evaluated in a small number of trials in adults, focusing on quite extreme forms of undesirable behaviour, such as coprophagia, verbal perseverations, which are far less likely to be seen in normal or high functioning adults (Bishop-Fitzpatrick 2016). While ABA may be effective in the highly specialised domains in which these behaviours occur, it has not been shown to have a role in attaining milestones associated in general, with adult life, such as increasing social interaction and relationship formation (Bishop-Fitzpatrick 2016).

Social skills training

Deficits in social, and particularly in non-verbal communication, skills, are a hallmark of autism into and beyond adulthood. A range of approaches are described in a recent overview (Laugeston and Ellingsen 2014). Unfortunately, the literature evaluating these approaches in adulthood is limited and not particularly encouraging.

We may also recall (in considering further research), that many patients on the autism spectrum describe learning to use these skills, but at a considerable cost in energy and effort. This may apply particularly to women (see earlier chapters), echoing the often heard remark, in the clinic, 'I've learnt how to fake it—but it's exhausting'. Such remarks often lead onto the discussion covered in the next chapter, on acceptance of an offering of reasonable adjustments to autism.

Genetic counselling

Occasionally, families ask about the risk of further family members being affected in the future. Counselling should precede any genetic testing (Tantam 2012), exploring the person's expectations and the implications of any result. To date there has been no evidence of approaches that can be recommended. Heritability of autism and autistic traits is high compared with mental and behavioural disorders and this can be pointed out to families. However, the mechanisms of inheritance are complex and there is no way of saying (or more to the point predicting) how future offspring may be affected. Rapin (2011) also argues that the complex nature of inheritance makes prenatal diagnosis and counselling unlikely to be feasible, for now.

Treatment of comorbidities

The topic of comorbidity management is discussed in this and in the next two chapters. For example, a central point for the psychiatrist, treating a mental disorder such as depression or psychosis, on realising that autism is also present, will be the need to reformulate the problem and the management plan, including making reasonable adjustments for the presence of autism. The psychiatrist, who has followed a course of learning for which this book is a guide, will already have two advantages to offer to their patient: one, a clear separation and identification of the autism and non-autism components of the patient's condition; and two, the ability to discuss and fully acknowledge each of these to the patient. Often that may be the most that can be done, but patients with such needs can find this level of understanding and consideration very helpful.

Here, we focus on treatment of people with autism, who also have psychiatric morbidities. In general, in principle, treatments that are effective for *anxiety, depression, psychosis,* and other comorbidities, should also work in adults with autism. However, perhaps surprisingly, as we shall now see, these treatments have yet to be evaluated objectively in this population. Knowing the patient also has autism may prevent harm, even if it does not bring measurable additional relief.

Pharmacotherapies for comorbidities

Arguments for caution with the use of pharmacotherapy have been discussed above. As an articulate patient with autism might well say, 'our brains are different, doctor—how can you be sure they will react in the same way to drugs that work on the brain? They could make things worse …'

In saying that, established treatments 'should work', we must also temper this with caution, acknowledging that we do not know that the harm benefit balance is the same in, for example, the treatment of depression in an autistic patient. If a patient reports back that they have been depressed for many years and different antidepressants have been tried, and nothing works, we should probably take that more seriously than we might in other patients. The most up to date advice by Research Autism (http://researchautism.net/) of the place of antidepressants in treating anxiety, or depression, in the presence of autism, also questioned whether we know what is their value: up to this point we still do not know.[6]

Psychotherapeutic approaches

Given all the arguments already marshalled in this book, the case for using psychological therapies ought to be a strong one also. However, again we still do not have an evidence base to help us.

A second problem is that providers of therapies may express reluctance to offer their services, saying that they do not know enough about autism to be able to work with such patients (for example, to treat depression).

Some observations come to mind from seeing patients and discussing the treatment of their psychiatric comorbidities with psychotherapists, including those treated before the autism component was recognized. Patients on Cognitive Behaviour Therapy (CBT) programmes are strikingly diligent in carrying out homework tasks. However, such patients struggle with group-based interventions and often have to drop out. Patients struggle with

---

[6] The interested reader could look at the detailed descriptions of the few trials of pharmacotherapy reported on adults.

describing emotions. Patients are prone to very concrete interpretations of what therapists say—this is quite challenging if the therapist does not realise at the time that autism underlies this.

There is a growing literature on how to approach psychotherapy of comorbidities in the adult on the autism spectrum (Anderson and Morris 2006; Gaus 2016).

Evaluating evidence in the future

Some existing compounds, used for other indications in neurology or for mental disorders, might also be put forward for evaluation in relation to core symptoms of autism. According to clinical trial registration a pharmaceutical compound is being evaluated in adolescents with autism, the primary endpoint being change from baseline in Vineland—II Adaptive Behavior Scale Composite Standard Score at Week 24.[7] A small controlled trial of Repetitive transcranial magnetic stimulation (rTMS) has reported a reduction on the social relatedness subscale of the RAADS compared with sham rTMS (Enticott et al. 2014). Hopefully, given such investment and effort, there will be something worthwhile to report on within the next 5–10 years.

New psychological approaches may also be forthcoming. For example, cognitive training or remediation, might be a fruitful future avenue for research on treatment effectiveness. A small number of studies have found that children with attention deficit hyperactivity disorder (ADHD) and children with autism also have an auditory processing disorder (APD; McArthur 2009). A child is said to have APD if she, or he, scores poorly on a test that asks them to detect, identify, discriminate, order, group, or localize sounds (McArthur 2009). Auditory training programmes have been suggested for treatment of specific language impairment, autism, and ADHD symptoms, in children (McArthur 2009). If these were to prove effective in children, it is possible that they might be evaluated in adults, as an initial open study indicates (Eack et al. 2013). Doubts about this approach have been expressed.[8]

The European Union (EU) Medicines agency has consulted on draft guidance on the development and evaluation of treatments in autism, which is likely to become a key benchmark, used by intervention developers,

---

[7] https://clinicaltrials.gov/ct2/show/NCT02901431

[8] Dawes P, Bishop D (2009) Auditory processing disorder in relation to developmental disorders of language, communication, and attention: a review and critique. International Journal of Language & Communication Disorders, 44: 440–465; Moore DR, Ferguson MA, Edmondson-Jones AM et al. (2010) Nature of Auditory Processing Disorder in Children. Pediatrics, 126: e382–e390.

including pharmaceutical companies. This is an important resource, as it also points to statutory and governance frameworks to be followed in trials within the EU. This document was put out for consultation before our group published its evaluation of outcome measures in clinical trials in autism (Brugha et al. 2015). One of our recommendations is that any trials conducted could also be used as an opportunity to evaluate (and develop) outcome measures specific to this population.

Legal aspects of the psychiatry of autism and of risk behaviours

Earlier reference was made to duties of the psychiatrist under law (Chapter 10) to give advice in relation to key issues such as depriving an adult of their liberty and in relation to *advising on mental capacity*. In Chapter 14 the issue of reasonable adjustments in relation to court proceedings is discussed.

There is increasing expectation that psychiatrists will consider autism in advising on legal matters just as they have always done in relation to mental illness. An introduction to this topic can be particularly recommended, which also addresses the advice that Courts may request for example in relation to criminal charges (Berney et al. 2014). In order to advise the courts on significant matters (whether civil or criminal), it is important to have a good level of experience and knowledge of autism, and this will amount sometimes to a significant degree of specialisation in the area, depending on the seriousness and complexity of the issue and potential consequences for the concerned individual.

There are a number of forms of disability associated with autism that may complicate the assessment of mental capacity and thereby the validity of an individual's consent to treatment. They include difficulties with comprehension, attention, and concentration, inflexible ways of thinking about how the world works, with coping with change, and difficulties or reluctance in coming to decisions. Comorbidities such as intellectual disability and ADHD may add to the complexity of assessment in such matters. These factors are discussed elsewhere in this book.

Most individuals with autism are keen to stay away from trouble (and indeed from the wider social world) and do not offend. We do not have firm evidence on whether adults with autism pose more or less risk to others than do the rest of the adult population.[9] However, adults with high risk

---

[9] If one works in the criminal justice area it is easy to gain the impression that autism is associated with increases in behaviours that are harmful to others. Unfortunately

behaviours, who may also have autism, are more likely to be referred to services and seen by psychiatrists. They may, therefore, require an assessment and management of risk that is informed by a knowledge and understanding of autism. There are a number of factors that may offset their law-abiding respect for rules and result in a vulnerable individual who is predisposed to getting into trouble. These include the following: a naive interpretation of social relationships, a misinterpretation of rules with a failure to appreciate social rules, difficulty in reading social signals, passivity leading to vulnerability to being exploited, impulsivity (which may be in part due to comorbid ADHD), a lack of awareness of the consequences of their actions, fascinations, and overriding preoccupations, which can lead to offences such as stalking, misjudging the nature of an interview leading to incautious frankness, for example in relation to private fantasies, and an inflexible failure to understand and to accept the need for change (Berney et al. 2014). These factors have also been discussed and described elsewhere in this book.

Education

It is surprising that the topic of education receives so little attention although arguably the training provided could lead to lasting benefits, thus meeting with our general definition of treatment. In the next two chapters the value of supporting adults through education and training receives consideration.

Conclusion

Opportunities for treatment that influence the course of autism in adulthood appear to be limited and disappointing. The widespread presence of autism throughout adulthood may be an impetus to developing safe effective treatments. This does not mean that we have nothing to offer to our patients now. In the Chapters 13 and 14 social care approaches at the individual, the family (and carer), and at the societal level are considered. The criteria for judging whether to use these are different from those applied to treatments.

---

the necessary representative general, and custodial, population (epidemiological) studies have not yet been completed and published, although suitable methods for conducting such research are available.

Chapter 13

Social care, the personal passport, and reasonable adjustments

Introduction

Much of the material in this chapter should be familiar to those clinicians who have had extensive experience of services in old age psychiatry as well as in community and rehabilitation psychiatry, in the last decade. Therefore, much of this chapter is aimed at the psychiatrist or clinical psychologist who has only detailed clinical experience in hospital and clinic psychiatry settings. The aim throughout Part III of this book is also to help a psychiatrist, who has not had training in autism, or who has not had a dialogue with someone they know has the condition, to see the world of autism as someone with the condition sees it, and to know how to help such patients. Therefore, for clinicians with considerable experience of community and social care practice, but who are unfamiliar with autism, the descriptions of the adjustments recommended in this chapter for autism may also have some value.

Social care ... What is it?

As medical students, and as trainee psychiatrists, this question often arose. In most settings treatments were tried first. Failing that, other therapeutic interventions may have been tried. However, if none of these worked, the role of medicine and therapeutics seemed to fade away. Somehow, others took over (sometimes, if not always). It is what one does next when treatment options are insufficient, or non-existent. It is common sense. In societies that do not have sophisticated social care systems, it is the doctor saying to the family, *'take him home, and take care of him. I can do nothing more'*.

A revolution in facing up to disability and giving society responsibility for accepting it, as a responsibility, is gradually taking over. In modern, rapidly industrializing societies, where adult children must often leave rural areas to seek employment in cities, it is the care, if any, that replaces the role that the family—the offspring in this case—can no longer supply.

However, the story of autism is 'upside down'. First, it is the child turned adult who cannot cope, and it is the older generation of parents, left to continue to support their adult offspring, as if (s)he were still a child. It is also upside down because autism is invisible. In some cultures, where disability brings shame on a family, the doctor might even have said, 'hide him away', which in the case of autism is a mistake because no one can see what is wrong and what can be done to help the person.

The family may say, 'something is wrong. He(she) is not showing independence. Brothers and sisters are doing fine, why not him'. They will often ask: 'Who will take care of him when we're gone?'

Support, not treatment, is now to be considered. It is about a different kind of service. It is not remedial (although the possibility of remedy should never be totally abandoned). In high income countries, it will be seen to be about tiers of services—with social care sometimes separate from health care, as in much, but not all of the United Kingdom—and sometimes integrated, if seemingly almost invisible, within or alongside of health services.

It is crucial for the clinician, learning about this, to accept the guidance of those with extensive experience of social and community care, to lead them forward, including being guided by social workers. In this way one learns that there are (or should be if adequately funded) systems in place, generally referred to as social care, which, now that a diagnosis has been made and a disability rendered visible, may have value within a parallel structure that previously might have been little understood. That is a structure accustomed to caring for other groups needing care—the elderly, children whose families cannot (or will not) care for them, and adults with major physical or mental impairments (for example victims of head injury, adults with moderate to profound intellectual disability). An example relevant to the isolated young adult with autism (possibly labelled 'Asperger syndrome') might be a social club dedicated to supporting young adults with the same condition.[1]

Effectiveness and social care

How do we know social care works? Where is the evidence base? What do we mean by effectiveness/helpfulness of social care? How do we judge it? What does effectiveness mean? This is rather akin to asking does a wheel

---

[1] In the city of Leicester, where the author developed an autism diagnostic service for adults, such a social club was also established in the late 1990's known as the 'Monday Club' (http://www.themondayclub.co.uk/).

chair work for someone who is paralysed from the waist down. Try removing it and you'll soon discover. The same general principle applies, although the need is less visible, less obvious, and sometimes you don't actually know if there is need until you remove the support. Therefore, when assessing a young adult, still living with family who does not wash, do housework, open official correspondence until prompted to by their parent/carer, how do we know if that care that the family are providing is needed? Often we don't until, in similar 'controlled' circumstances, we try and see what happens when support is removed. Clearly, a thoughtful approach to understanding and evaluating social care is needed.

What are the specific objectives of social care for the adult on the autism spectrum? Given an adult with significant social communication problems what would care be?

At the time clinical diagnostic services for adults were beginning to develop, agencies that were working with adults with autism and intellectual disability, were beginning to give consideration to the idea that similar approaches might be helpful to the more able adult with autism, who is not intellectually disabled—that was also known then as Asperger Syndrome. A second example, at about the same time, was the setting up of another support group for parents with adult offspring, known as the 'Asperger Syndrome Support Group', which was also a voluntary organization (sometimes referred to as the 'third sector').

Personal choices

Personal choice is of considerable importance. We are talking here about adults who are free to make choices about the help that may be on offer. Many would say no to offers of help. Their carers would then, possibly, have to face the challenge of pointing out that they cannot live there, forever. More often than not such patients have already figured that one out—'but as it's not a problem today', 'spending the day on the X-box or Playstation', or whatever technology, in their bedroom, just seems like a nicer prospect.

It is about knowing what your condition is, how you differ from others. Most adults in this population have some degree of awareness that they have always been different and don't really fit in. See again the example of Case Study F, in Chapter, 2, the young adult with a background of being isolated at school and 'not fitting in'.

The value of learning about how they differ from most others—neurotypicals—is sometimes not such an obvious next step. Some do and they embrace the difference. Andal in her book on self-diagnosing autism (Andal 2015) also suggests that, once the person has decided that they have autism (whether self identified or officially diagnosed), they should consider each of their traits in different day to day contexts, how much impact they have now and how to cope with them if they are a challenge.

In the clinic, following a diagnosis, patients are encouraged to attend sessions run by a local autism charity, designed to discuss the diagnosis and what it means and what help and support is available locally for them, should they choose it. This means discussing their situation with others in the same position. A carer is also encouraged to take part in this kind of opportunity. The role of carers and their needs will be addressed at the end of this chapter. Parents and local charities have also developed and maintained an invaluable list of local organizations and agencies that list such sources of informal and formal support.

Reasonable adjustments

A key concept in this society, in relation to acknowledging and supporting persons with disabilities, is the concept of reasonable adjustments. It is now illegal for a large public building not to have access points, adjusted for people with mobility problems, hearing difficulties, blindness, etc. Autism is now embedded in that legislation (taken up in the next chapter).

The concept of the Personal Passport[2] has also been developed to assist in describing what someone with a disability needs help and adjustments for. A first step is to enable the person with autism to consider, as part of a social care assessment, 'How do I prefer you to understand me?' Assessment results must be from the patient perspective. (S)he needs a profile for others to work with that reflects what they want, as much as need. This is also a journey of discovery and learning, which should be accommodated and embedded in the modes of social care assessment used in that community or society.

To take a concrete example, people on the autism spectrum also need to attend clinics and hospitals. A hospital passport sets out the adjustments needed for accessing a hospital and related clinical settings, physical, psychiatric, and other, taking account of the nature of autism and how it affects a person's functioning. Given the nature of autism, that must mean that staff know, before the patient arrives, that this patient has autism and that we need some understanding of what that means and how to *communicate* clearly and effectively (without the staff member feeling, perhaps, that this is a very rude person). The next chapter picks up on the societal implications of this insight. It will often mean that noise is a crucial issue and that artificial lighting and

---

[2] Also known as a hospital passport or a communication passport.

even smells may be important—if we are not, in effect, to exclude such patients from environments they need to access occasionally.

Reasonable adjustments need to be made by us, psychiatrists, and by fellow mental health professionals. This may be awkward, because it is our job and our role to recognize and know how to deal with all manner of mental and behavioural variations from the normal. As we know from earlier chapters, may not we have been so good at that. It is our job to enable the triggering of the processes of labelling that enables recognition, reasonable adjustments, and personal (or communication) passports. This right is enshrined in a society in disability rights—in UK law—and in the USA in the Americans with Disabilities Act (ADA, 2008; see next chapter).

The personal passport

Until a couple of years ago a written 'personal passport' was only seen in services for adults with an intellectual disability. Now there is a smartphone App called AutisMe that is freely available for android and apple operating systems for smart phones (see Apple Store or Google). AutisMe is designed to give users the space to express their personality, to create and change the way they want to be seen, understood and helped. It allows the person to create a list of the things important to them, as well as keeping important information about their needs, and space to keep their emergency contacts.

Social care services for adults on the autism spectrum

Social workers are the lead social care profession in autism, as in many other areas of disability.[3] Built into their training and professional ethos is *an acceptance of how things are,* akin to the philosophy underlying palliative care, and philosophically distinct from medical treatment approaches that emphasize recovery. Social workers are also adept in several key ways: assessment of needs not met by treatment, liaison with other services across a broad range, including education, housing, welfare, healthcare, criminal justice systems, etc. Increasingly, their historical role as sources of social support and counselling, has been overtaken in publicly funded settings and structures by a *brokerage role*, identifying individual need, identifying resources to meet need, developing a care plan and implementing and monitoring it over time, as mentioned earlier.

---

[3] This role would be led by a nurse in areas of physical disability.

> **Box 13.1 Working options and contexts within the wider care system and autism needs**
>
> - Supporting families that can care.
> - Embedded in mental health services.
> - Working with adult safeguarding procedures.
> - Supporting physical health services from primary care to hospital care.
> - Working with welfare and benefits systems.
> - Further and higher education and educational (dis)ability support teams.
> - Housing agencies and officers.
> - Employment support and supported employment.
> - Leisure and recreation services including reasonable adjustment showings in cinema and theatre, and other areas, such as gyms and swimming pools.
> - The charitable, voluntary, and third sectors.
> - Liaising with the criminal justice system, legal advisers, and probation (parole) officers.
> - Other social agencies, such as charities, faith communities, and clubs devoted to activities and interests.

Adults on the autism spectrum are vulnerable and open to exploitation in many ways, organizationally, discriminatory, monetary, physical, emotional, through neglect, because of self-neglect, through modern slavery, domestic abuse, sexually, and are also vulnerable to their freedoms being restricted. The protection of vulnerable adults, therefore, is also part of the role of social workers (and of other agencies such as the police); vulnerable adult *safeguarding procedures*, which do exist, often parallel those set up to protect children.

In summary, the role of the social worker is one of working with and within other systems, making use of available resources. We will now consider these in terms of examples (Box 13.1) in the context of autism in adulthood and later years.

Family support

Perhaps, the most important structure in society that social workers work with, is still the family, where there is still a family, which is in a position to provide some level of support. In traditional, and in some low and middle income (LMIC) societies, that may, indeed, be the only form of social care available. The principles are similar to those applying to families caring for a member with any long-term disability such as, for example, a child with intellectual (learning) disabilities, a parent with cognitive decline and, perhaps, growing frailty. The person cared for often prefers it (it is essential that their views are considered). Perhaps, because of their values, the family may also prefer it. However, it must not be allowed to become unsustainable. Respite care is sometimes made available, although mainly for the autistic adult with some degree of intellectual disability (or learning difficulties). For families to support effectively, they also need to be supported.

Working with the system—the value of working with social workers embedded in mental health service teams

During almost four decades of working within the NHS in England, the author has seen two periods in which social workers were employed outside the health system, by local authorities, and two in which they became part of the mental health team, under a single team manager (who often was an experienced social worker). It has seemed that when social care staff are part of the mental health service system that the most rapid advances have been made in relation to developing autism social care. These advances include 'awareness raising' within mental health teams, assessment appropriate to need, appropriate treatment and care, and training of staff across disciplines. Although psychiatric services sometimes exclude adults on the autism spectrum as 'not for us', this is less likely when a social worker with autism training is an active team member, able to contribute views and alternative perspectives and share responsibility.

In recent years, policy has directed social workers, and community care agencies, to support adults with disabilities, such as autism, to make their own choices with support allowances, sometimes termed 'personalized budgets'. The care client, in effect, can make his or her own choice, to spend a cash allocation on their chosen form of care, such as a support worker, or on some other source of support they decide will help them cope with their disability. This bold move in policy has yet to be evaluated in terms of cost effectiveness and the satisfaction or dissatisfaction of adult service users with autism. Anecdotal accounts range from the satisfied client who has always wanted this freedom, the client who is still denied any control over expenditure on their own care, to the distressed and perplexed adult on the spectrum told that if they pay a care worker they are now an employer with the duties and responsibilities that entails.[4]

In the community, the coordination of risk management will often involve the social worker (unless major risks are being managed that involve the criminal justice system; see also the subsection on Advice to the courts). Interventions may be aimed at changing the social environment (for example, who the person lives with) when problems are identified offering help, such as advice to the family, partner, or carer(s), and suggesting changes or accommodations to the physical environment. Psychosocial interventions for higher risk or challenging behaviour, which should involve additional input from other mental health team professionals, such as psychology or psychiatry, should include: clearly identified target behaviour(s); a focus on outcomes that are linked to quality of life; assessment and modification of environmental factors that may contribute to initiating or maintaining the behaviour; a clearly defined intervention strategy; a clear schedule of reinforcement, and the capacity to offer reinforcement promptly and contingently on demonstration of the desired behaviour; a specified time scale to meet intervention goals (to promote modification of intervention strategies that do not lead to change within a specified time); a systematic measure of the target behaviour(s) taken before and after the intervention to ascertain whether the agreed outcomes are being met (NICE, 2012).

Working with the system and welfare benefits

Even in settings, systems, and societies, where there is no acknowledgement of the existence of autism, in otherwise able adults, there are other systems in society that can be worked with to further the interests of such adults. Criteria used in deciding on allocation of welfare benefits often cover the needs of persons on the autism spectrum. These include difficulty in obtaining and holding down paid employment for health reasons. Social workers (and or family carers), with some determination, can help an adult on the autism spectrum to obtain the welfare benefits to which they should be entitled.

---

[4] Giving an adult on the autism spectrum such additional responsibilities in law may be imprudent and even psychologically harmful as they may lack the capacity to deal with such responsibilities.

Working with the system and further education programmes

Many more advanced societies have developed support arrangements for adults in education, to ensure that success in completing a course is not hampered by health problems or disability. There is no reason why an adult cannot be supported with the subtle, but sometimes quite disabling cognitive and communication impairments that can come with having autism. Within the past decade, autism (or 'Asperger syndrome'), became a specified disability on the application form for universities and higher education institutions, in Great Britain, even before knowledge of its existence was becoming as widely known as it now is.

The availability of funded resources through local education authorities has sometimes been a lifeline for a student with autism; previously, many such students 'dropped out' within the first semester (or term), due to inability to cope with the many demands of college or university living, including the social demands and the expectations of living independently and caring for oneself. A few specialist further education colleges also exist that make specific provision for autism, but individual students may have to fail to cope with main stream education, due to complexity and fragility, before they can seek a place at such a specialist college.

Housing, employment, and occupation

As we shall see in the next chapter, these are also areas in which society is endeavouring to recognize and adjust to the needs of adults with autism. Because of the ways employment and housing related organizations are taking note of and adapting to autism, social workers are less closely and intensively involved than they were in the past. Societal adjustment to autism, in author's view, is the way forward (Chapter 14). Many examples were included in Chapter 4, on the perspective of people with autism in the work place.

Supported employment might have more enduring effects beyond a support function. As stated earlier, executive function improvement was shown in a supported employment trial of Garcia-Villamisar and Hughes (Garcia-Villamisar and Hughes 2007). An overview of employment and ASD suggests that supported employment programmes promote job placement, satisfaction, and retention (Howlin et al. 2005; Gerhardt et al. 2014).[5]

---

[5] Chapter 4 on the perspective of the person with autism includes a detailed discussion of difficulties in the employment setting and how with acceptance and training so much seems more achievable.

Advice to the courts on reasonable adjustments within criminal justice processes

A key issue is ensuring that reasonable adjustments are made so that the adult involved in legal proceedings can follow what is happening and understand legal procedures. Within this, a common problem is where the autistic adult is subject to questioning, or interrogation, without the presence of a responsible adult, who understands their disabilities. Similar issues apply to the adult with intellectual disability, but the adult with autism who is otherwise functioning at a higher level may not be considered to require adjustments unless this is pointed out. Social workers and probation officers and services have a key role to play in recognition and support of adults on the autism spectrum, in order to ensure justice. The advice of the psychiatrist can carry considerable authority. Advice may include pointing out that an adult with autism, if testifying, may behave in a manner that misleads the court into thinking that they have no feelings or concerns about the effects of their behaviour. They may also have difficulty in the cognitive processing of information and evidence and in advising their lawyer and may, therefore, need longer periods of time in order to be able to take part effectively.

Other contexts for social care

It is helpful to advise GP's to keep autism in mind, when making referrals to hospitals and other health services, to ensure that reasonable adjustments will be made, something that might not arise until many years following a diagnostic assessment.

Other contexts, to be considered in the wider community, include leisure and recreation facilities. For example, increasingly, the development of commercially provided cinema showings, dedicated to the autism population, are developing (and indeed the subject of autism is being included with increasing sophistication within the plot lines of movies). Social workers and indeed other support workers, should seek out these kinds of opportunities and encourage their development in communities that are still falling behind in this regard.

Other social agencies, such as charities, faith communities, clubs devoted to activities and interests, and services for homeless adults

There are also other settings that can play a role that is in concert with their values. Faith communities can often play a crucial role in helping with social isolation. They need to be encouraged to learn more about autism, its recognition and the most effective ways of communicating with and of supporting such persons in their communities. This also applies to organizations, whether voluntary or statutory, that support the most isolated adults in our communities, such as those who are homeless.

Occupational therapy

Occupational therapists can become involved in the assessment of an adult whose autism has not until then been recognized. Their role is ideally placed to speed up awareness recognition and assessment. There is limited experience of their role with the more able adult with autism. For example, they could, perhaps, have a role in assisting employers to make reasonable adjustments on behalf of an employee on the autism spectrum.

Carers needs

Carers also have needs; it can be an enormous plus to find people who have had to cope with the same issues in their offspring, or partner, to pass on lessons to others and to learn from them. A *carer's needs assessment* is the duty of health and social care systems, within the NHS, with a clear pathway being published and sustained for each community and service area.

Conclusion

In the next chapter we will shift the focus to the wider community and society, and ask what more can be done to make adjustments to the needs and the potential, of people on the autism spectrum. Some readers may be wondering why a psychiatrist is suggesting this—arguably it is within our potentially influential public health and public mental health role, with attendant leadership opportunities and responsibilities. Whereas Chapter 13 has been orientated towards addressing the individual person's needs for social care for the adult with significant autism spectrum disorder, Chapter 15 will take the wider societal perspective and could be viewed as of interest also to policy makers, planners, commissioners, who will turn to psychiatrists and other clinicians for advice and sometimes leadership.

Chapter 14

Caring communities and caring societies

Background

Given that autism is largely an untreatable disorder, at present, for which adjustments need to be made by others in order to enable a good and productive quality of life for adults with the condition, the wider community and society have a role to play. As reviewed in Chapter 1 current best estimates, based on epidemiological prevalence surveys in England, suggest that 1 in 100 adults are significantly affected. The combination of several adult surveys from our research team, suggest that approximately 1 in 3 of these adults is classed as long-term disabled and not seeking employment. Health economic projections (based on older estimates of the burden that are being revised) argue strongly for investment in employment support that should give a positive return economically (Buescher et al. 2014).

In this chapter, we reflect on the role of society and link that back to the personal, individual level, already considered in the previous chapter. Policy, evidence, relevant sectors, and stake holders are considered, and we will again look at specific contexts where society can improve life quality in the key sectors of housing, education, employment, etc. In any society, when formulating policy and when planning, the advice of psychiatrists is likely to be sought, for example, by interpreting epidemiological information and its implications for society beyond 1:1 clinical practice. In the same way it may also serve public health intelligence, and health needs assessment, considerations. Therefore, this chapter is also relevant and important to psychiatrists.

Policy development

How does a caring society, or a region or district, use clinical and epidemiological information in the interests of adults with autism, and their carers, and the services that are expected to identify and meet their needs? Who are the key wider stake holders, in policy, in planning, in commissioning, in public provider services, and in businesses that may be setting out to provide services? In many countries policy on autism does not even come into consideration in the way that expenditure is budgeted for. Government action on autism and the impact of population research on policy has been greatest in a growing number of States of the US, and in the nations of the UK. Government Policy on autism is also developing elsewhere in Europe. Policy in these two countries has been influenced by two contrasting ways of counting how many people have autism (Brugha 2016).[1] The community survey case finding method (Appendix 1) has led to the informed conclusion that in England autism affects approximately 7 per 1000 adults (and a similar proportion of children (National Institute for Health and Clinical Excellence (Great Britain) 2012; Hill et al. 2016).

Examples of policy development in the US and the UK may be helpful. Until now a key difference between these two national systems has been that, in the UK, treatment is free at the point of use (funded from central taxation) and, although it is only free in exceptional cases, social care is provided through local government authorities, who levy local taxes to support their duties. The US insurance-based system is also beginning to allow for payments for the social causes of health outcomes, as in public funding for social care: https://www.openminds.com/market-intelligence/executive-briefings/roi-addressing-social-determinants-health/?utm_source=OPEN+MINDS+Circle&utm_campaign=3487782cc1-EMAIL_CAMPAIGN_2017_01_09&utm_medium=email&utm_term=0_eecbede49c-3487782cc1-160612537. However, the future of US health and social care policy development is less certain at the time of writing.

In the United States, a key obstacle to assisting people, beyond childhood, has been the widespread experience across most states of mandating treatment within childhood only. It is widely acknowledged and constantly echoed, in the comments of parents, that when you reach that upper age limit (varying from 18 to approximately 21 years) you 'fall off a cliff', meaning that there is nothing there to support the young adult.

The US Presidential Candidate, Mrs Hillary Clinton, published online in January 2016 a policy on 'Community Supports and Services for Individuals Transitioning into Adulthood' (https://www.hillaryclinton.com/briefing/factsheets/2016/01/05/hillary-clintons-plan-to-support-children-youth-and-adults-living-with-autism-and-their-families/). The Clinton policy referred to 'the landmark 1999 ruling in Olmstead v. L.C. that codified the right under the Americans with Disabilities Act (ADA) for individuals with disabilities to live in the community rather than institutions, and

---

[1] Appendix 2 sets out some of the experiences of the author in government policy development.

to gain access to reasonable accommodations to support their independence'. Furthermore, it was pointed out that 'since passage of the ADA Amendments Act of 2008, people with autism have received the ADA's protections against discrimination in employment, government services, public accommodation, and other kinds of discrimination.' A pledge was made to 'launch a new Autism Works Initiative consisting of a postgraduation transition plan for every student with autism aging out of school-based services and a public-private partnership with employers that is designed to grow to include hundreds of firms over time'. A range of policies for adults were included, covering Savings accounts, support to care givers, and employment. A specific recommendation was to ensure access to assistive technologies: 'for children and adults with autism who struggle with verbal communication, assistive technologies can help them better communicate with others and achieve greater independence. These tools can range from communication books and picture boards to iPads and text-to-voice devices'.

Information was also a key part of the policy programme with a call for:

'the first-ever adult autism prevalence and needs study. While the Centers for Disease Control has long measured the incidence of autism in 8-year old children, no comprehensive study of the prevalence and needs of autism in adults has been conducted in the United States. When the United Kingdom conducted an adult prevalence survey, they learned valuable information regarding the needs of adults on the autism spectrum that has helped them craft and improve services. Clinton will instruct the CDC to conduct the United States' first-ever population level survey of adults on the autism spectrum'.

At the time of writing, it is unclear what policy for autism is being developed or might be enacted by a new US Government, from 2017 onwards. It is worth pointing out that, in general, there has been little if any evidence of partisanship in the development of national policies in relation to autism and disability (in contrast to aspects of general health policy).

Clinton referred to policy development in the United Kingdom, building on adult survey information. An Autism Act (2009; http://www.legislation.gov.uk/ukpga/2009/15/contents) was passed by parliament with all party support. An autism strategy was developed (there are separate similar arrangements for each of the four nations of the United Kingdom). There are two broad indications that the design of the policy has been influenced by the survey information (the collection of which was funded from central government). In the United Kingdom there is no other condition or disease with its own Act of Parliament.

First, it makes specific recommendations for older adults and those past working age. This would have been unheard of until it was demonstrated by the survey programme that autism is approximately as common in older adult life as in younger adulthood and, indeed, in childhood (albeit the precision of these estimates is not as satisfactory as one would wish).

Second, it is also cross-sectoral—in some ways not unlike the aforementioned US policy proposals—with specific actions being put in place across many different central and local government departments. Thus, in addition to health and local authority social care (which has led responsibility in England for care, following an autism diagnosis in adulthood), the policy for England extends to government departments responsible for the criminal justice system, education, welfare benefits, housing, and employment.

The Autism Act also binds the most senior health minister in England, the Secretary of State for Health, who sits in Cabinet, to report annually to parliament on progress with the implementation of the objectives of the Act.[2]

The European Union takes some Europe wide responsibility for certain aspects of public health—most health policy being led nationally and not at the EU level. Information and support for policy development for autism is supported by the EU. *Link* is the newsletter, which brings together examples of good practice and accounts of progress towards national policy development (http://www.autismeurope.org/files/files/link-65-en.pdf). Policy development and implementation varies considerably between European regions and countries.

Policy implementation

At the time the policy in England was being developed, there was a widespread assumption that all adults with autism had very high levels of disability and need. The lifetime cost of addressing this had been estimated to be $2.2 million per adult in the UK, and $2.4 million in the USA (Buescher et al. 2014), which is clearly unaffordable, if all adults estimated to have autism have such high levels of need. Clearly, more precise information on levels of disability is required before there is any point in revising these projected estimates. An affordable solution is needed.

The second challenge was getting care to people with autism and to their carers, where there are high levels of care needed. Given finite resources, and limited prospects of increased funding, alternatives to expanded funding

---

[2] This work has been supported by an Autism Programme Board, of which the author has been an active member, meeting under the chairmanship of a government health minister three times per year.

were needed in order to achieve parity of provision across all conditions including autism.

Public workforce retraining

Experience with planning began in a few forward thinking localities and in some it was recognized that the first step to take was to train the existing health and care workforce to be aware of autism as an issue throughout the life course. Training programmes to retrain the care workforce were developed. This book (Chapters 2 and 3 in particular) reflects elements of that retraining, but targeted at adult psychiatrists. The components of the training were to raise awareness and to equip the professional to communicate effectively with the person with autism, and to support them to access and make use of resources used by other disability groups. Apart from the cost of training there were no new up-front costs. The effect was to begin to reduce the exclusion from care services of adults whose condition was autism rather than another disability or a mental health condition.

This retraining strategy is not an unusual or original solution. It had positive impacts in local areas engaging in it (until funding cut backs to local authority care teams in the mid-'twenty-teen' years set us back). Training of professionals, organizations, carers, even the affected persons themselves seemed to have a crucial role. Differences between social and health care professionals, including values, standards, approaches, were taken into consideration in developing training materials.

Implementation of the Autism Act has brought about similar changes more widely. The national policy identified front line teams in each administrative sector and required them to undergo basic training—again, on awareness raising and on basic strategies for more effectively supporting such adults to access services (such as housing, welfare benefits, support to enter employment, and make full use of educational and training courses, etc.). For example, in many areas police officers have been given basic training. In clinical practice, in a growing number of cases, a referral for an autism assessment of an undiagnosed adult was triggered by a public employment officer asking a client had they considered this as a possible reason for often losing a job. Job loss often occurred within a short time of commencing a new work role. Lawyers, magistrates, and judges would increasingly make similar suggestions where they suspect autism might be a factor in offending behaviour, or might at least be a factor in determining the support such a person may need.

There are many other strands to the policy for England, which can be viewed through government reports and guidance documents (Department of Health 2010, 2015). More contentious has been the extent to which government was willing to require certain departments, particularly health, to target funding growth to adults with autism and to diagnostic teams. This is an ongoing challenge. However, compared with previous decades and to other parts of the world the amount of progress made is striking.

Autism also began to be specified in revisions of many relevant legislative provisions, such as for example in a revision to mental health legislation that is called into use when compulsory detention of adults with severe mental illness requires consideration. Advocacy organizations, notably the National Autistic Society, played a major part in pressing for the necessary changes.

Service sector industry and charities and third sector organizations have also become involved. There are growing, but still anecdotal accounts, that large food and department stores now seek to recruit and train, and support, adults on the autism spectrum to work in their store ware house areas, because such persons follow instructions very precisely and reliably. Similar anecdotal accounts come from employers of technical and engineering staff. The value to an employer of technically able individuals on the autism spectrum is not over looked.

Evaluating the effectiveness of the implementation of policy on autism

Accordingly how is the effectiveness of such a policy to be objectively evaluated? The answer to this question also takes us back to the need for key knowledge and skills, which are possessed by professionals identifying and supporting people with the condition. There are several components to this.

As we know from Chapter 1 autism became one of the conditions covered in the regular seven yearly programme of Adult Psychiatric Morbidity Surveys (APMS) beginning in 2007 (which is before the policy had been developed—a fortuitous information baseline). There has since been a second survey in 2014, showing essentially no significant change in prevalence and little change in the numbers of adults with autism in receipt of mental health care (suggesting that a lot more work still needs to be done).

The second component is known as the Autism Self Assessment Framework (SAF), which builds on similar data collection on services for people with intellectual disability (https://www.gov.uk/government/publications/autism-self-assessment-framework-exercise). Data collection takes place within local authorities for their areas approximately 18 monthly. Topics reported upon include all the examples mentioned above including support in each area (housing, employment, etc.), areas covered in commissioning, the development of diagnostic centres and their current waiting list lengths and waiting times, the establishment of a local planning and or autism local 'partnership board' etc. Each authority is required to involve people with autism alongside authority officials in completing the SAF returns to verify their authenticity.

Other programme implementation evaluation exercises include visits to localities and local health boards by officers from central government, accompanied by advisers drawn from professionals and advocates with autism expertise.

Population needs assessment and public health surveillance

Planning for services also requires a process for quantifying need through needs assessment programmes and through the use of monitoring and surveillance programmes. The APMS is limited in what it can provide, in part because it is not ideal for tracking service activity regularly and when policy implementation is at an early stage of development.

The Centre for Disease Control (CDC) and Prevention in Atlanta has developed a surveillance programme that tracks activity and, in particular, recognition of autism, by periodically sampling and evaluating educational and health records in 8-year-old children (Centers for Disease Control and Prevention 2012). The programme shows increases in recognition over the years since the programme began, which if just reflecting recognition is pleasing, but of concern is that recognition rates vary to an extreme degree from one area to the next within the USA (Hill et al. 2016). This suggests that there could be over counting in some areas and, of particular concern, considerable and continuing under-recognition in other areas, all of which suggests great difficulty in establishing consistent benchmarks for diagnosis between areas. This programme has also been frequently mistaken for being an epidemiological prevalence (or incidence) programme, which clearly it cannot be (Brugha et al. 2014; Brugha 2016). Inconsistency in applying diagnostic thresholds for autism in adults has also been shown in our own validation work (Brugha et al. 2012). This is one of the reasons why the use within population surveys of precise and consistent case finding methods is the only basis for estimating population prevalence (Brugha, 2016) (Brugha et al. 2014).

Third sector and/or charitable involvement in policy and implementation

Before leaving this topic we need to consider briefly, which sectors should be considered in the development and implementation of policy, throughout the process of implementation and evaluation. Any such policy development process should ask the question, who else needs to be involved? The area of autism is characterized quite strikingly by its strong national societies (the National Autistic Society (NAS) in the UK, Autismspeaks (USA), Autism Europe, etc.), which have driven policy and service development to an unusual extent. The Autism Programme Board for England has included family members with experience and carers and persons with the condition, educational and other governmental organizations, policy-makers representing employment (but oddly not employer representative organizations), internal affairs (the Ministry for Justice and the Home Office in England) covering police, probation, and criminal justice systems, and the welfare benefits systems. Each of these areas of policy influence, development and implementation can draw attention to tensions within the system and, by communicating through a health minister, can lead to rapid action through communication between relevant government ministers. When legislation is being updated these links can ensure that opportunities are grasped to improve the legal framework, supporting adults on the autism spectrum.

Chapter 15

Choices in life, and the awareness, knowledge, and skills to support them

The importance of training

Before writing this book there was no suitable background source that adult psychiatrists could turn to in order to help them develop knowledge, understanding, awareness, and a capacity to develop skills and clinical experience with adult autism. Together with Drs Tom Berney and Peter Carpenter, and assisted by many others, training programmes were developed under the auspices of the Royal College of Psychiatrists in London and the Irish College of Psychiatry in Dublin. To date, apparently there are no similar courses mounted and led by our profession elsewhere.

Whether by coincidence, or because of other initiatives, and because of growing public understanding and interest in autism across the life course, there is the impression that this training is beginning to have an impact. Referrals by adult psychiatrists to autism diagnostic clinics have grown strikingly in recent years, and many of their patients did not know they had, or might have, autism. Previously referrals were triggered by knowledgeable families and general practitioners. It would be a positive outcome if this book was successful in enabling such continuing professional development to be taken to scale more widely.

Because of the nature of autism and experience of teaching the subject to many different professionals, the strategy has been adopted of setting the subject out from multiple different perspectives in the hope that everyone reading it will find a viewpoint or perspective that works for them, that captures their interest and concern. Feedback would be very welcome.

Autism for too long has been taken for granted as a childhood condition for child health, child mental health, and educational professionals to deal with on behalf of all society. We now know this is falsely restrictive. The condition affects adults approximately equally across the life span. It impacts on all walks of life. We all need to share in it some interest, concern, and indeed as professionals, responsibility.

Of all of these many perspectives, it is that of the person with autism (or autistic traits) that deserves our particular attention. Importantly, the language that patients with autism have used to present their viewpoint has also been included where it seemed to add meaning and understanding (see in particular Chapter 4). An unexpected realization, during the same period that this book was being written, has been the extent to which adults can describe quite clearly most aspects of autism, as it affects them, when interviewed using carefully constructed, searching questions (see in particular Chapter 8). The practice of restricting adulthood assessment of autism to childhood assessment (albeit retrospectively) and to direct behavioural observational approaches, may need to be reconsidered. As we know, in the older adult a valid source of information on early development will not be available often. Opportunities to observe an adult communicating and functioning also seem to be more limited than would be the case with children (Chapter 9) because of the possibly distorting effect of significant psychiatric comorbidities. If adults can be shown, with the help of refinements in interviewing methods, to provide a valid account of their autism (as has happened with the assessment of ADHD in adulthood), there are greater prospects of improved and more precise outcome assessments for use in autism clinical trials and prevalence surveys. This would enable us to begin to develop the science base for knowledge and treatment of autism in adulthood that is so clearly lacking, which is so evident in what it has been possible to include in this book.

Gaps in the evidence base and future research priorities

We have also talked about prospects for the future. The field until recently has been marked by a great deal of optimism that 'magic bullet', clinically applicable solutions (see Chapter 3, final footnote) would be found through genetic and neuroscience research, that there would be a clear biomarker test, and that there would be one or more treatments that transform the condition. This has not happened. If anything we are realising that autism is (or perhaps the autisms are) far more complex than can be tackled in this way. Laboratory researchers need to be cautious in the assumptions they make in phenotyping the participants in their research so that their work on biomarker tests will be relevant and may bring 'early wins'.

Although more remote on the translational pathway to the clinic and the community, there continues to be the need for biological and other more fundamental forms of research, particularly on a topic such as autism that seems to be the most 'brain based' of all the conditions psychiatrists work with. Currently, topical areas one could mention include the gut microbiome or the role of oxytocin, as examples of potential biological mechanisms and pathways. The author's personal 'gut feeling' is that breakthroughs will be more likely to come from less expected 'left stage' angles, such as from fundamental breakthroughs in our basic understanding of brain chemistry and biology. We still know very little about how brains work. Understanding the brain in autism is likely to require a basic understanding of brain processes. For example, this might come through work on insects and fish, the simplest brain forms known to us, that permit the ethically acceptable, experimental manipulation of social and communication behaviour with far more rapid results, thus accelerating hypothesis falsification (Popper 1963) and verifiable scientific progress.

What one would hope and look forward to is that autism recognition in childhood will grow as it clearly is doing in a few fortunate areas, and that this knowledge will follow the child through transition into adult care, through services, understanding, and acceptance, within the very different world of adulthood, in which families are no longer able to continue to provide levels of protection and support they naturally give in childhood. We are beginning to see exciting evidence of at least one breakthrough in the development and testing of the long-term benefits of a very early childhood intervention that may possibly continue to have a positive benefit beyond childhood (Pickles et al. 2016). That promising achievement was based on slow, painstaking work, carried out diligently and patiently over many years.

In the Preface and throughout this book, the limited research evidence available to guide practitioners has been openly acknowledged. Preparing this book has helped to highlight the many gaps in evidence. What are the clinical (translational end stage) research priorities for autism in adulthood? The nosological status of autism remains unclear in relation to other forms of neurodevelopmental delay. Epidemiology may be able to contribute to answering this; clinical researchers need to keep this in mind in choosing what to measure and how. Epidemiology has yet to be harnessed satisfactorily to study psychological, social, cultural, and environmental factors associated with the course and outcome of autism throughout adulthood. Assuming autism (or the closely interconnected 'autisms') endure, with descriptive definitions close to those that have evolved up to now, work is needed on tests to identify those more likely to need an assessment, and on assessment methods. Such measures need to be compatible with adult and older age groups, where early developmental information may not be available to collect. Outcome measures for clinical trials need to be developed and evaluated that cover core autism features, associated features, comorbidities, and especially those outcomes that matter to people with autism and their carers. Trials are needed that answer questions such as, which adults benefit from having an assessment and a diagnosis (such trials would include people suspected to have, but are then found not to have autism); these kinds of studies probably need to be conducted in different age groups because what is good for a young adult may be unnecessary or even harmful for an older adult. One would also hope to see the development and use, in adequately powered, large scale treatment trials, of well validated adult outcome measures of both core autism and associated non-autism outcomes, with which people with the condition want help. Clearly, there are aspects of having autism that bring difficulties, if not to all, then to many adults on the autism spectrum, and therefore we need interventions, treatments, including medications, that address effectively and safely these core autism symptoms. The same applies to comorbid conditions that affect some people with autism. We do not know if conventional treatments for depression or anxiety are effective, safe, and relevant. Research is also needed on longer-term outcomes starting in early adulthood with follow-ups to the years beyond normal retirement age.

Learning needs—reflecting and looking forward

Before ending, and (as always follows at the conclusion of a training event), we need to review our learning needs and plan for the future. We also need to consider further reading options. The Royal College of Psychiatrists in London has proposed a list of learning needs for doctors and psychiatrists at the level of general medical training, general psychiatric training and the training of psychiatrists with a recognized specialist expertise in psychiatry (Berney et al. 2006), and Table 15.1.

Experience also points to several needs that run in parallel with this, which may need separate emphasis.

First, as we learnt when looking at referral and at initial assessment, adults coming for an assessment may have complex and, not necessarily, clear reasons for being there. Other people close to them may also have a critical role leading up to a decision to undertake an assessment. Following a diagnosis other people close to them may also have a critical role in building on the potential benefits of recognition. As a psychiatrist both of these factors require skill, confidence, expertise, in dealing with more than just the one patient (Table 15.1). Partners may be involved. Parents and other first degree relatives, such as an older sibling, may be involved. Therefore, experience

Table 15.1 Competencies expected of a non-specialist adult psychiatrist

Topic	Chapters in this book
Knowledge	
Demonstrate a working knowledge of the alerting signs and the clinical features of autism in the adult with ability in the range from mild intellectual disability through to high functioning levels.	2 and 3
Have a basic understanding of the core deficits in autism and the implications of these for the adjustment and care of individuals and their families.	3, 12, and 13
Be able to describe the causes and development of autism and appraise newly emerging research findings (learning objectives for psychiatrists)	1, 3, and 12
Skills	
Have the ability to communicate with and relate effectively to a person with autism and to their family, partner, carers.	7 and 8
Be able to take a developmental history from a parent, suitable older relative or other appropriate informant (and to recognise the pointers to these disorders).	3 and 7
Experience	
Have the opportunity to interview, assess, and treat people with autistic-spectrum disorders under an experienced supervisor (learning objectives for psychiatrists in the early stages of postgraduate training).	7–10, and 12

Source: data from: Berney et al., CR136. Psychiatric services for adolescents and adults with Asperger syndrome and other autistic-spectrum disorders, Copyright 2006, Royal College of Psychiatrists.

gained in a good psychiatric training programme in working with couples and families can be invaluable and, indeed, may play an important part in achieving a good assessment outcome and a good post diagnostic plan for support and adjustment, in the longer term.

Audit and professional peer group activities are an important underpinning to the role of the clinician engaging in assessment. A useful example could be an audit of local referrals by adult psychiatrists seeking assessments that focuses in retrospect on the evaluation of need for that assessment (see Chapters 5 and 6).

Recommended general and further reading

There are three recent volumes (Amaral et al. 2011; Tantam 2012; McDougle, 2016), which cover the nature of autism and its underpinning research. Research literature in this area is rapidly growing. Therefore, these are recommended as a starting point for the reader, who should search for more recent developments on topics that may require particular action.

The first of these volumes is by a single author who has covered a large literature single handedly (Tantam 2012). The author is a clinician, a psychiatrist, and a psychotherapist, with an extensive knowledge of the underpinning neurosciences. Furthermore, the author covers childhood and notably also adulthood. As such this volume has an unusual degree of coherency and consistency.

The second of these is a multi-contributor overview of the research literature (Amaral et al. 2011). Although many of the authors are not involved in clinical practice this has not limited its value to practitioners. It gives hardly any attention to autism beyond childhood because most research on autism involving human participants is only on children.

The third most recent volume is designed to address the background reading needs of clinicians (McDougle 2016). Most chapters address the condition in childhood and three also address aspects of autism as it affects adults. Chapters also include case studies, for the most part in childhood. An excellent chapter, cited in the present volume, summarizes the latest literature on the epidemiology of autism in childhood. Some of the chapter authors are engaged in clinical practice.

Amaral, D., Dawson, G., and Geschwind, D.H. (2011) Autism spectrum disorders. New York: Oxford University Press.
McDougle, C.J. (2016) Autism Spectrum Disorder. New York: Oxford University Press.
Tantam, D. (2012) Autism Spectrum Disorder throughout the Lifespan. London: Jessica Kingsley.

The topic of autism in adulthood is now beginning to receive some attention. There are many books on various aspects of practical approaches to helping people with autism. Two that stand out are multi-author works covering autism, respectively, in adolescence and adulthood (Volkmar et al. 2014) and in mid- and later life (Wright 2016).

Volkmar, F., Reichow, B. and McPartland, J.C. (2014) Adolescents and Adults with Autism Spectrum Disorders. New York: Springer.
Wright, S.D. (2016) Autism Spectrum Disorder in Mid and Later Life. Philadelphia: Jessica Kingsley.

For an overview of what works in autism, albeit mainly in childhood but also where evidence is available in adulthood, which is based on a constantly updated website resource, is Flemming and his colleagues second edition of a comprehensive book on autism interventions.

Flemming, B., Hurley, E., and Mason, J. (2016) Choosing Autism Interventions: a research-based guide. Hove: Pavilion Publishing and Media Ltd.

There have also been useful authoritative overview articles on the topic of autism in prestigious medical journals, such as the Lancet, in recent years that are recommend for short, quicker introductions although, again, there is relatively little in these on autism in adult and later life (Wing 1997; Levy et al. 2009; Lai et al. 2014; Lancet (Editorial) 2016).

Lai, M.C., Lombardo, M.V., and Baron-Cohen, S. (2014) Autism. Lancet **383**, 896–910.

Lancet (Editorial) (2016) Pride in autistic diversity. Lancet **387**(10037), 2479.

Levy, S.E., Mandell, D.S., and Schultz, R.T. (2009) Autism. Lancet **374**, 1627–1638.

Wing, L. (1997) The autistic spectrum. Lancet **350**, 1761–1766.

Appendices

Appendix 1
Epidemiology methods

This section provides details of adult epidemiological research methods used to generate the findings on adults set out in Chapter 1.

To answer the question, how many adults have autism, the method used should count everyone with the condition, and not just those whose condition has been diagnosed and recorded. Given that autism is a new condition that was completely unrecognized, except in highly specialized settings until the end of the twentieth century, it was all the more important that the method of identification was not reliant on information collected by services. This required the development of case finding methods that can be deployed feasibly, and cost effectively, in health surveys in random samples of the whole population, untreated and treated (Brugha and Meltzer 2008).

Epidemiological methods in autism have developed as understanding and recognition has developed, i.e. slowly and unsurprisingly, until recently, only in studies of autism in childhood. Methods for studying the epidemiology of mental and behavioural disorders in populations have also developed slowly with major survey programmes only getting underway in the 1990s (Robins and Regier 1991; Kessler et al. 1994; Jenkins et al. 1997).

The research design then being used for counting mental disorder rates (and factors associated with them) was a two phase survey design. In phase one of the APMS, lay interviewers used structured questionnaires to collect information on symptoms of mental disorders and associated factors, from a random sample of adults throughout the survey area (in the first survey, in 1993, the areas covered were England, Wales, and Scotland, excluding the Highlands and Islands). As with the assessment of psychosis, in the APMS surveys, the ADOS (module 4) was used in phase two of the survey. In 2007 618 ADOS interviews were completed and in 2014–5 a further 629 ADOS assessments (APMS 2014; http://content.digital.nhs.uk/article/3739/national-study-of-health-and-wellbeing) were completed in randomly sampled adults, living in private households in the community, throughout England. See also Appendix 2 and 4 for further background information.

A totally different method, known as surveillance, for keeping track of changes in rates of a disease over time, showing a trend for increased reporting of autism in childhood over time, has been highly influential in public debate in the USA (Centers for Disease Control and Prevention 2012). It has led to growing pressure on the USA to mandate autism coverage. Until now there has been no research in the USA in adults on rates of autism (see Chapter 14). State autism mandates apply only up to the end of childhood (as early as age 18).

Appendix 2

The author's experiences in epidemiology and in policy development

The author spent a period of 18 months working as a mental health policy Senior Medical Officer at the Department of Health in London, in the mid-1990s. While there it was realized that until autism was studied epidemiologically in adults, in the same way as psychosis and common mental disorder, there was little likelihood of official government policy interest and tangible financial input to the topic of autism in adults (in spite of considerable lobbying by quite vocal autism charities). A search was begun for evidence of such research, but none was found. Experts were contacted, including the childhood autism epidemiology expert Eric Fombonne, in Montreal. Eric confirmed the results of these initial researches.[1]

Autism posed new challenges to this survey method, the greatest being that at that time the 'diagnosis' of autism depended largely on evaluating information on the course of development from early childhood, with particular emphasis on social communication through non-verbal and verbal language. Within such a survey approach, obtaining information from parents or directly from survey respondents themselves, on development at least 15 years previously was not realistic.[2]

With the survey programme designer, the epidemiologist Howard Meltzer, methods for measuring psychosis in such surveys had been adapted from clinical research interviewing methods. In a second survey phase, psychosis was assessed in approximately 1 in 10 of those who had completed the

---

[1] Eric also added a remark that greatly encouraged me to try harder. He added 'and if anyone does do such a survey I think it will be you'.

[2] An expert group meeting in the USA concluded at about the same time that a survey of adults could not be done or, at least, viable methods for doing so did not exist.

first phase of interviews. Psychosis was assessed using the survey version of the World Health Organisation Schedules for Clinical Assessment in Neuropsychiatry (WHO SCAN; Wing et al. 1990). The ADOS was chosen as an approach that got around the problem of assessing autism in an adult without having to collect collateral information; it is administered directly to a child or adult by a trained clinician. In other words the ADOS approach could work within the adult survey two phase design. It had never been used in this way before. Further information on its evaluation is included in Appendix 4.

Amongst the researchers contacted then was the autism research psychologist Simon Baron-Cohen, at the University of Cambridge. Simon had been carrying out a survey of children, with the help of the Cambridge public health specialist, Carol Brayne, using complex sampling techniques that included random sampling in schools and evaluations of children who were already coming to the attention of services. Simon introduced the author to a post-doctoral researcher at Cambridge, Fiona Scott, who had worked with Simon and Carol on their Cambridge autism childhood survey. Fiona was then one of the most experienced users and trainers in the Autism Diagnostic Observational Schedule (ADOS; Lord et al. 1994), which they were using in their survey.

Dr Scott trained the author's team in the ADOS, and helped with thinking through whether the ADOS might need to be adapted or altered in any way to work with older and elderly adults, living independently in the community, without being able to speak to a carer, relative, or any other informant. We came to the conclusion that no changes needed to be made to the ADOS ratings, but that the kinds of questions and probes used might need to be adapted to the context of a community living, older adult (until then the ADOS was being used from pre verbal child hood through to young adulthood, in the context of referrals to and assessments carried out in specialist autism clinics).

However, in order to conduct a survey with the ADOS in the community, credibility and acceptance, and one's own confidence in any findings, would depend on work cross validating the method against more conventional and generally accepted ways of assessing autism that include the assessment of childhood development (Chapters 3, 7). All of these issues were seen as having direct application to the development of assessments in clinical practice (of direct relevance to the purposes of this book). The validation work designed with my research collaborators and then carried out with my research team and with five other experienced clinical diagnosticians (three clinical psychologists and three consultant psychiatrists) is explained in technical detail in work completed before any epidemiological findings were published (Brugha et al. 2012). The results of these initial findings based on the third Adult Psychiatric Morbidity Survey in 2007 (APMS; Brugha et al. 2011) were based on cross validation work, including a modified ADOS scoring algorithm, similar to, but not precisely the same as the original ADOS algorithm used in clinical populations (Lord et al. 2002), further described in Appendix 4.

Funding was also obtained to conduct a supplementary survey, using as the sampling frame adults with intellectual disability, listed on population case registers in three parts of England. With this the estimates of rates of autism across the able adult community and adults with intellectual disability (from moderate to profound levels of impairment) could be combined (Brugha et al. 2016).

Appendix 3

Development of a new approach to interviewing adults about their experiences of autism based on the Schedules for Clinical Assessment in Neuropsychiatry (Chapter 8)

Chapter 8 is possibly the most 'experimental' or 'provisional' of this book. The best known and most widely used autism assessment method used in current practice in adults is the ADOS. The ADOS is primarily designed to elicit examples of communication and social interaction behaviour. However, in general, it does not include detailed questions about symptoms of autism in the way that a psychiatric psychopathology interview does. Doing so would represent a departure from autism assessment methods used up to that time. Therefore, the author and collaborating colleagues, Dr Tom Berney of the University of Newcastle and Dr Peter Carpenter, Bristol, have been developing a systematic approach to the assessment of autism based on, and reliant upon, a direct interview with the patient in the adult psychopathology tradition.

The principle underlying this approach is familiar to adult psychiatrists. It rests on the supposition that an adult (or an older child), who is experiencing the effects of a mental disorder, can provide an account of their experiences and perceptions to someone willing to interview them. (Historically the alternative option was to base judgements as to a person's mental state on observations of their behaviour, an approach that still dominates the assessment of younger children and intellectually disabled adults).

The current published version of the SCAN interview (version 2.1 at the time of writing) covers the major mental disorders seen in adulthood, including complex disorders such as psychosis, mania, and obsessive compulsive disorder, where some element of clinical judgement is needed by the interviewer. Each section of the SCAN interview includes instructions on time periods to be covered in that part of a SCAN interview, which correspond with what is known of the time course of the syndromes and disorders being covered.

The current and previous versions of the SCAN do not cover developmental disorders.[1] Nor does the SCAN cover personality disorders, but an example of a similar method for assessing personality disorders that shares the same semi-structured, investigator rated, approach is the International Personality Disorder Interview (IPDE; Loranger et al. 1994). Both the SCAN and IPDE have been used in a study in the Netherlands of adults seen at an autism assessment clinic, compared with a larger group seen in general mental health clinics (Ketelaars et al. 2008). The SCAN approach has also been extensively used in international cross cultural and epidemiological studies.

This new SCAN neurodevelopmental disorder section is being developed, also, with the support of other experienced SCAN developers and trainers, who have limited experience of assessing adults with autism. For them such a development would need to integrate clearly and meaningfully with current and past versions of the SCAN approach to assessing common and severe forms of psychopathology, found in adults under the care of psychiatric services.

This new additional development of the SCAN interview that is currently being evaluated by the SCAN development group incorporates sub-sections covering both autism and ADHD, as they present in adulthood. Chapter 8 makes use of relevant aspects of this new approach to set out how an interview can be used to evaluate autism symptoms, or autism 'psychopathology'. The approach to interviewing about symptoms of ADHD is not as novel; there are currently two adult ADHD semi-structured interviews used in research (DIVA; CADID; Ramos-Quiroga et al. 2016), but neither of these two semi-structured interviews includes glossary definitions and rating

---

[1] An exception to this is an autism checklist and a number of observational ratings that may indicated the presence of autism.

guidance on each symptom covered (although training does provide such guidance).

A direct interview approach is much needed, particularly for evaluations in older adults in whom the methods described in Chapter 7 are not feasible, because of the lack of information on development in childhood. Preliminary experience of interviewing patients using this new SCAN Neurodevelopmental section is promising, at the time of writing.

This approach to training is also being used in the form of a training interview, now published and available to download, developed by us under the auspices of the Royal College of Psychiatrists, which has apparently been quite popular (http://www.rcpsych.ac.uk/pdf/asperger_interview_use_this_one.pdf), and which is currently being updated to reflect the DSM-5 criteria for autism.

In Chapter 10, on the assessment of comorbidity, a unique objective of this addition of neurodevelopmental disorder to the SCAN, will be explained—in effect a method for differentiating symptoms that could be due to either autism or a mental disorder (or occasionally both), which has always been part of the SCAN approach.

Unfortunately the full revised WHO SCAN interview is not available for distribution at the time of writing, but it should be not long after this book is published. It is hoped to have this extended version of the SCAN (tentatively designated as version 3), available for others to use, to learn and evaluate independently during 2018 or 2019, following the anticipated publication by WHO of ICD-11.

Appendix 4

Independent evaluation of the ADOS in community populations

A training programme for interviewers on Module 4 of the Autism Diagnostic Observational Schedule (ADOS-4) was developed, according to ADOS principals (Lord et al. 2002), using typical examples of abnormal behaviours likely to be encountered in adults living in the community (Brugha et al. 2012). Volunteers assisting in the training usually had a clinician determined diagnosis of ASD. There was little difficulty in discussing, and agreeing on, ADOS-4 ratings, when considered in the context of independent adults living unsupported in the community. For example when rating 'Quality of Social Overtures', which is a rating of the quality of the respondent's attempts to initiate social interaction with the examiner, it is stated (Lord et al. 2002) that 'special attention should be given to the form of the overture and its *appropriateness to the social context*' [italics added].

Algorithms for autism spectrum disorder and for autism are incorporated in the ADOS-4 (Lord et al. 2002). Selected ADOS-4 ratings that correspond to DSM-IV and ICD-10 criteria for Pervasive Developmental Disorders (PDD) are summed to a total score for Communication and Reciprocal Social Interaction, to which two thresholds are applied, for non-specific PDD (7 or greater on the ADOS-4 combined total score: termed ADOS 7+) and for Autism (10 or greater on the ADOS-4 combined total score: termed ADOS 10+). In the author's research, similar algorithms have been used, after conducting two evaluative studies, partly in order to calibrate the optimal threshold score to use (Brugha et al. 2012). The ADOS is only one component of a diagnostic assessment, which should include information from an informant (Lord et al. 2002).

Survey field work interviewing did not commence until the team of four survey interviewers was achieving at least 90% agreement on ratings of jointly observed ADOS-4 examinations. Total scores on the ADOS were compared with two reference points: a diagnosis of autism on the DISCO (described in Chapter 7), based on further interviews with carers; and the opinions of experienced clinicians, given access to detailed information from the national community survey, on a range of individuals including those thought to have autism. Although agreement between the clinicians was poor, their modal threshold ratings corresponded closely to those provided by the DISCO assessments and, with the recommended threshold for the Module 4 ADOS total score, originally developed in a clinical population. Prevalence rates were only published (Brugha et al. 2011), when this calibration work had been completed (Brugha et al. 2012).

References

Aman, M.G., Singh, N.N., Stewart, A.W., and Field, C.J. (1985) The aberrant behavior checklist: a behavior rating scale for the assessment of treatment effects. American Journal of Mental Deficiency **89**, 485–491.

Amaral, D., Dawson, G., and Geschwind, D. H. (2011) Autism spectrum disorders. New York: Oxford University Press.

American Psychiatric Association (2013) Diagnostic and Statistical Manual of Mental Disorders, 5th edn (DSM-5™). Washington DC: American Psychiatric Press.

Andal, L. (2015) AM I AUTISTIC? A Guide to Autism & Asperger's Self-diagnosis for Adults. London: New Idealist Ltd.

Anderson, S. and Morris, J. (2006) Cognitive behaviour therapy for people with Asperger syndrome. Behavioural and Cognitive Psychotherapy **34**, 293–303.

Argyle, M. (1978) Non-verbal communication and mental disorder. Psychological Medicine **8**, 551–554.

Argyle, M. (1987) Bodily Communication. London: Methuen and Co.

Arnold, L., Aman, M., Martin, A., Collier-Crespin, A., Vitiello, B., Tierney, E., Asarnow, R., Bell-Bradshaw, F., Freeman, B., Gates-Ulanet, B., Klin, A., McCracken, J., McDougle, C., McGough, J., Posey, D., Scahill, L., Swiezy, N., Ritz, L., and Volkmar, F. (2000) Assessment in multisite randomized clinical trials of patients with autistic disorder: the autism RUPP network. Journal of Autism and Developmental Disorder **30**, 99–111.

Ashwood, K. L., Gillan, N., Horder, J., Hayward, H., Woodhouse, E., McEwen, F. S., Findon, J., Eklund, H., Spain, D., Wilson, C. E., Cadman, T., Young, S., Stoencheva, V., Murphy, C. M., Robertson, D., Charman, T., Bolton, P., Glaser, K., Asherson, P., Simonoff, E., and Murphy, D. G. (2016). Predicting the diagnosis of autism in adults using the Autism-Spectrum Quotient (AQ) questionnaire. *Psychological Medicine.* **46**, 2595–2604.

Asperger, H. (1944) Die autistischen Psychopathern im Kindersalter. Archiv für Psychiatrie und Nervenkrankenheiten **177**, 76–136.

Asperger, H. (1991) 'Autistic psychopathy' in childhood. In: Autism and Asperger Syndrome (ed. U. Frith), pp. 37–92. Cambridge: Cambridge University Press.

Baird, G., Simonoff, E., Pickles, A., Chandler, S., Loucas, T., Meldrum, D., and Charman, T. (2006) Prevalence of disorders of the autism spectrum in a population cohort of children in South Thames: the Special Needs and Autism Project (SNAP). Lancet **368**, 210–215.

Baron-Cohen, S. (1985) Does the autistic child have a 'theory of mind'? Cognition **21**, 37–46.

Baron-Cohen, S., Scott, F.J., Allison, C., Williams, J., Bolton, P., Matthews, F.E., and Brayne, C. (2009) Prevalence of autism-spectrum conditions: UK school-based population study. British Journal of Psychiatry **194**, 500–509.

Baron-Cohen, S., Wheelwright, S., Robinson, J., and Woodbury-Smith, M. (2005) The Adult Asperger Assessment (AAA): a diagnostic method. Journal of Autism and Developmental Disorders **35**, 807–819.

Baron-Cohen, S., Wheelwright, S., Skinner, R., Martin, J., and Clubley, E. (2001) The autism-spectrum quotient (AQ): evidence from Asperger syndrome/high-functioning autism, males and females, scientists and mathematicians. Journal of Autism and Developmental Disorders **31**, 5–17.

Baxter, A.J., Brugha, T.S., Erskine, H.E., Scheurer, R.W., Vos, T., and Scott, J.G. (2015) The epidemiology and global burden of autism spectrum disorders. Psychological Medicine **45**, 589–600.

Bech, P. (2013) Autism as the clinical core marker in schizophrenia. World Psychiatry **12**, 81.

Berney, T., Adamou, M., Brugha, T., Faruqui, R., Carpenter, P., Kalinidi, S., Le Couteur, A., Milton, D., Mukaetova-Ladinska, E., Swinton, M., and Tantam, D. (2014) Good practice in the management of autism (including Asperger syndrome) in adults, College Report CR191. In: (ed. Royal College of Psychiatrists), p. 36. London: Royal College of Psychiatrists. Available at: http://www.rcpsych.ac.uk/usefulresources/publications/collegereports/cr/cr191.aspx (accessed 29 July 2017).

Berney, T., Brugha, T., Carpenter, P., Curran, M., Davies, S., Holloway, F., Kearney, S., Le Couteur, A., McCulloch, C., Moriarty, J., Roy, M., Sivagamasundari, U., Staufenberg, E., and Tantam, D. (2006) Psychiatric services for adolescents and adults with Asperger syndrome and other autistic-spectrum disorders. In: Good practice in the management of autism (including Asperger syndrome) in adults (ed. Royal College of Psychiatrists), p. 39. Royal College of Psychiatrists: London.

Berument, S., Rutter, M., & Lord, C. (1999). Autism screening questionnaire: diagnostic validity . British Journal of Psychiatry, **175**, 444—451.

Bilder, D., Botts, E.L., Smith, K.R., Pimentel, R., Farley, M., Viskochil, J., McMahon, W.M., Block, H., Ritvo, E., Ritvo, R.A., and Coon, H. (2013) Excess mortality and causes of death in autism spectrum disorders: a follow up of the 1980s Utah/UCLA autism epidemiologic study. Journal of Autism and Developmental Disorders **43**, 1196–1204.

Bishop-Fitzpatrick, L. (2016) Psychosocial interventions and community-based services for adults with autism in the United States. In: Autism Spectrum Disorder in Mid and Later Life (ed. S. D. Wright), pp. 323–332. Philadelphia: Jessica Kingsley.

Bishop-Fitzpatrick, L., Minshew, N.J., and Eack, S.M. (2013) A systematic review of psychosocial interventions for adults with autism spectrum disorders. Journal of Autism and Developmental Disorders **43**, 687–694.

Bodfish, J.W. (2011) Repetitive behaviors in individuals with autism spectrum disorders. In: Autism Spectrum Disorders (eds D. Amaral, G. Dawson, and D. H. Geschwind), pp. 200–212. New York: Oxford University Press.

Bodner, K.E., Beversdorf, D.Q., Saklayen, S.S., and Christ, S.E. (2012) Noradrenergic moderation of working memory impairments in adults with autism spectrum disorder. Journal of the International Neuropsychological Society **18**, 556.

Brugha, T. (2016) Autism and ageing. Epidemiology and demographics. In: Autism Spectrum Disorder in Mid and Later Life (ed. S. D. Wright), pp. 334–344. Philadelphia: Jessica Kingsley.

Brugha, T.S., Doos, L., Tempier, A., Einfeld, S., and Howlin, P. (2015) Outcome measures in intervention trials for adults with autism spectrum disorders; a systematic review of assessments of core autism features and associated emotional and behavioural problems. International Journal of Methods in Psychiatric Research **24**, 99–115.

Brugha, T.S., McManus, S., Bankart, J., Jenkins, R., Smith, J., and Scott, F. (2014) The proportion of true cases of autism is not changing. BMJ Clinical Research Edition **348**, g3774.

Brugha, T.S., McManus, S., Bankart, J., Scott, F., Purdon, S., Smith, J., Bebbington, P., Jenkins, R., and Meltzer, H. (2011) Epidemiology of autism spectrum disorders in adults in the community in England. Archives of General Psychiatry **68**, 459–465.

Brugha, T., McManus, S., Meltzer, H., Smith, J., Scott, F.J., Purdon, S., Harris, J., and Bankart, J. (2009) Autism Spectrum Disorders in adults living in households throughout England—report from the Adult Psychiatric Morbidity Survey 2007. Leeds: NHS Information Centre.

Brugha, T.S., McManus, S., Smith, J., Scott, F. J., Meltzer, H., Purdon, S., Berney, T., Tantam, D., Robinson, J., Radley, J., and Bankart, J. (2012) Validating two survey methods for identifying cases of autism spectrum disorder among adults in the community. Psychological Medicine **42**, 647–656.

Brugha, T.S. and Meltzer, H. (2008) Measurement of psychiatric and psychological disorders and outcomes in populations. In: International Encyclopedia of Public Health (eds K. Heggenhougen and S. Quah), pp. 261–272. San Diego: Academic Press.

Brugha, T.S., Spiers, N., Bankart, J., Cooper, S.A., McManus, S., Scott, F.J., Smith, J., and Tyrer, F. (2016) Epidemiology of autism in adults across age groups and ability levels. British Journal of Psychiatry **209**, 498–503.

Buescher, A.V., Cidav, Z., Knapp, M., and Mandell, D.S. (2014) Costs of autism spectrum disorders in the United Kingdom and the United States. JAMA Pediatrics **168**, 721–728.

Centers for Disease Control and Prevention (2012) Prevalence of Autism Spectrum Disorders—Autism and Developmental Disabilities Monitoring Network, 14 Sites, United States, 2008, p. 19. Atlanta: Centers for Disease Control and Prevention. Available at: https://www.cdc.gov/mmwr/pdf/ss/ss6103.pdf (accessed 29 July 2017).

Colman, A. (2001) Dictionary of Psychology. Oxford: University Press.

Colvert, E., Tick, B., McEwen, F., Stewart, C., Curran, S.R., Woodhouse, E., Gillan, N., Hallett, V., Lietz, S., Garnett, T., Ronald, A., Plomin, R., Rijsdijk, F., Happe, F., and Bolton, P. (2015) Heritability of autism spectrum disorder in a UK population-based twin sample. JAMA Psychiatry 72, 415–423.

Constantino, J.N. and Gruber, C.P. (2002) The social responsiveness scale. Los Angeles: Western Psychological Services.

Darwin, C. (1873) The Expression of the Emotions in Man and Animals. London: John Murray.

Davidson, C.J., Kam, A., Neeham, F., and Stansfield, A.J. (2015) No exclusions—developing an autism diagnostic service for adults irrespective of intellectual ability. Advances in Autism, 1, 66-78. Delargy, Y. (2013) Top tips for diagnosing, supporting and meeting the needs of people on the autistic spectrum. Leicestershire: Leicestershire County Council. Available at: http://www.heathlanesurgery.co.uk/website/C82121/files/Autism_top_tips_web%5B1%5D.pdf

Department of Health (2010) Fulfilling and rewarding lives: the strategy for adults with autism in England. London: Department of Health. Available at: http://dera.ioe.ac.uk/22991/1/autism-guidance.pdf (accessed 29 July 2017).

Department of Health (2015) Statutory guidance for Local Authorities and NHS organisations to support implementation of the Adult Autism Strategy. London: Department of Health. Available at: http://dera.ioe.ac.uk/22991/1/autism-guidance.pdf (accessed 29 July 2017).

Doyle, C.A., McDougle, C.J., and Stigler, K.A. (2014) Pharmacotherapy of behavioural symptoms and psychiatric comorbidities in adults with autism spectrum disorders. In: Adolescents and Adults with Autism Spectrum Disorders (eds F. R. Volkmar, R. Reichow, and J. C. McPartland), pp. 161–191. New York: Springer.

Dunn, J. (2004) Children's Friendships. Oxford: Blackwell.

Eack, S.M., Greenwald, D.P., Hogarty, S.S., Bahorik, A.L., Litschge, M.Y., Mazefsky, C.A., and Minshew, N.J. (2013) Cognitive enhancement therapy for adults with autism spectrum disorder: results of an 18-month feasibility study. Journal of Autism and Developmental Disorders 43, 2866–2877.

Enticott, P.G., Fitzgibbon, B.M., Kennedy, H.A., Arnold, S.L., Elliot, D., Peachey, A., Zangen, A., and Fitzgerald, P.B. (2014) A double-blind randomized trial of deep repetitive transcranial magnetic stimulation (rTMS) for autism spectrum disorders. Brain Stimulation, 7, 206–2011.

Feinstein, A. (2010) A History of Autism. Chichester: Blackwell.

Findling, R. L. (2005) Pharmacological treatment of behavioural symptoms in autism and pervasive developmental disorders. Journal of Clinical Psychiatry, **66**, 26–31.**Flemming, B., Hurley, E., and Mason, J.** (2016) Choosing Autism Interventions: a research-based guide. Hove: Pavilion Publishing and Media Ltd.

Freeman, B.J., Ritvo, E.R., Yokota, A., and Ritvo, A. (1986) A scale for rating symptoms of patients with the syndrome of autism in real life settings. Journal of the American Academy of Child and Adolescent Psychiatry **25**, 130–136.

Fyson, R. and Kitson, D. (2007) Independence or protection – does it have to be a choice? reflections on the abuse of people with learning disabilities in Cornwall. Critical Social Policy, **27**, 426–436.

Garcia-Villamisar, D. and Hughes, C. (2007) Supported employment improves cognitive performance in adults with Autism. Journal of Intellectual Disability Research **51**, 142–150.

Gaus, V. (2016) Psychotherapy with older adults on the autism spectrum. In: Autism Spectrum Disorder in Mid and Later Life (ed. S. D. Wright), pp. 193–205. Philadelphia: Jessica Kingsley.

Gerhardt, P.F., Cicero, F., and Mayville, E. (2014) Employment and related services for adults with autism spectrum disorders. In: Adolescents and Adults with Autism Spectrum Disorders (ed. F. R. Volkmar, R. Reichow, and J. C. McPartland), pp. 105–119. New York: Springer.

Gillberg, C. and Kadesjo, B. (2003) Why bother about clumsiness? The implications of having developmental coordination disorder (DCD). Neural Plasticity **10**, 59–68.

Gillberg, I.C. and Gillberg, C. (1989) Asperger syndrome—some epidemiological considerations: a research note. Journal of Child Psychology Psychiatry **30**, 631–638.

Goodman, W.K., Price, L.H., Rasmussen, S.A., Mazure, C., Delgado, P., Heninger, G.R., and Charney, D.S. (1989a) The Yale-Brown Obsessive Compulsive Scale. II. Validity. Archives of General Psychiatry **46**, 1012–1016.

Goodman, W.K., Price, L.H., Rasmussen, S.A., Mazure, C., Fleischmann, R.L., Hill, C.L., Heninger, G.R., and Charney, D.S. (1989b) The Yale-Brown Obsessive Compulsive Scale. I. Development, use, and reliability. Archives of General Psychiatry **46**, 1006–1011.

Gotham, K., Pickles, A., and Lord, C. (2009) Standardizing ADOS scores for a measure of severity in autism spectrum disorders. Journal of Autism and Developmental Disorders **39**, 693–705.

Gotham, K., Pickles, A., and Lord, C. (2012) Trajectories of autism severity in children using standardized ADOS scores. Pediatrics **130**, e1278–e1284.

Grandin, T. (2011) Top priorities for autism/Asperger's research: perspective from a person with autism. In: Autism Spectrum Disorders (eds D. Amaral, G. Dawson, and D. H. Geschwind), pp. 1377–1385. New York: Oxford University Press.

Green, H., McGinnity, A., Meltzer, H., Ford, T., and Goodman, R. (2005) Mental Health of Children and Young People in Great Britain, 2004. Palgrave McMillan: Hampshire.

Guy, W. (1976) CGI (Clinical Global Impression) In (Anonymous), DHEW NIMH: NIMH.

Happe, F. (2006) The Weak Coherence Account: Detail-focused Cognitive Style in Autism Spectrum Disorders. Journal of Autism and Developmental Disorders, **66**, 5-25.

Hill, A.P., Zuckerman, K., and Fombonne, E. (2016) Epidemiology of autism spectrum disorder. In: Autism Spectrum Disorder (ed. C. J. McDougle), pp. 181–204. New York: Oxford University Press.

Hirvikoski, T., Mittendorfer-Rutz, E., Boman, M., Larsson, H., Lichtenstein, P., and Bolte, S. (2016) Premature mortality in autism spectrum disorder. British Journal of Psychiatry **208**, 232-238.

Howlin, P., Alcock, J., and Burkin, C. (2005) An 8 year follow-up of a specialist supported employment service for high-ability adults with autism or Asperger syndrome. Autism **9**, 533–549.

Howlin, P., Savage, S., Moss, P., Tempier, A., and Rutter, M. (2014) Cognitive and language skills in adults with autism: a 40-year follow-up. Journal of Child Psychology and Psychiatry **55**, 49–58.

Iacoboni, M. (2011) The Mirror Neuron System and Imitation. In: Autism Spectrum Disorders, (eds D. Amaral, G. Dawson, and D. H. Geschwind), pp. 99–1009. New York: Oxford University Press .

Jenkins, R., Lewis, G., Bebbington, P., Brugha, T., Farrell, M., Gill, B., and Meltzer, H. (1997) The national psychiatric morbidity surveys of great Britain-- initial findings from the household survey. Psychological Medicine **27**, 775–789.

Jordanova, V. (2012) Suicidality in adults with Autistic Spectrum Disorders. Preliminary findings presented to the World Psychiatric Association Section on Epidemiology and Public Health 2012. Sau Paulo: Brazil.

Kanner, L. (1943) Autistic disturbance of affective contact. In: (Anonymous), pp. 217–250.

Kato, K., Mikami, K., Akama, F., Yamada, K., Maehara, M., Kimoto, K., Kimoto, K., Sato, R., Takahashi, Y., Fukushima, R., Ichimura, A., and Matsumoto, H. (2013) Clinical features of suicide attempts in adults with autism spectrum disorders. General Hospital Psychiatry **35**, 50–53.

Kessler, R.C., Adler, L., Ames, M., Demler, O., Faraone, S., Hiripi, E., Howes, M.J., Jin, R., Secnik, K., Spencer, T., Ustun, T.B., and Walters, E.E. (2005) The World Health Organization Adult ADHD Self-Report Scale (ASRS): a short screening scale for use in the general population. Psychological Medicine **35**, 245–256.

Kessler, R.C., McGonagle, K.A., Zhao, S., Nelson, C.B., Hughes, M., Eshleman, S., Wittchen, H.U., and Kendler, K.S. (1994) Lifetime and 12-month prevalence of DSM-III-R psychiatric disorders in the United States. Results from the National Comorbidity Survey. Archives of General Psychiatry **51**, 8–19.

Ketelaars, C., Horwitz, E., Sytema, S., Bos, J., Wiersma, D., Minderaa, R., and Hartman, C.A. (2008) Brief report: adults with mild autism spectrum disorders (ASD): scores on the autism spectrum quotient (AQ) and comorbid psychopathology. Journal of Autism and Developmental Disorders **38**, 176–180.

Krug, D.A., Arick, J., and Almond, P. (1980) Behavior checklist for identifying severely handicapped individuals with high levels of autistic behavior. Journal of Child Psychology and Psychiatry **21**, 221–229.

Lai, M.C., Lombardo, M.V., and Baron-Cohen, S. (2014) Autism. Lancet **383**, 896–910.

Lancet (Editorial) (2016) Pride in autistic diversity. Lancet **387**(10037), 2479.

Laugeston, E.A. and Ellingsen, R. (2014) Social skills training for adolescents and adults with autism spectrum disorder. In: Adolescents and Adults with Autism Spectrum Disorders, (eds F. R. Volkmar, R. Reichow, and J. C. McPartland), pp. 61–85. New York: Springer.

Le Couteur, A., Rutter, M., Lord, C., Rios, P., Robertson, S., Holdgrafer, M., and McLennan, J. (1989) Autism diagnostic interview: a standardized investigator-based instrument. Journal of Autism and Developmental Disorders **19**, 363–387.

Leekam, S.R., Libby, S.J., Wing, L., Gould, J., and Taylor, C. (2002) The Diagnostic Interview for Social and Communication Disorders: algorithms for ICD-10 childhood autism and Wing and Gould autistic spectrum disorder. Journal of Child Psychology and Psychiatry **43**, 327–342.

Levy, S.E., Mandell, D.S., and Schultz, R.T. (2009) Autism. Lancet **374**, 1627–1638.

Loranger, A.W., Sartorius, N., Andreoli, A., Berger, P., Buchheim, P., Channabasavanna, S.M., Coid, B., Dahl, A., Diekstra, R.F., Ferguson, B., et al. (1994) The International Personality Disorder Examination. The World Health Organization/Alcohol, Drug Abuse, and Mental Health Administration international pilot study of personality disorders. Archives of General Psychiatry **51**, 215–224.

Lord, C., Petkova, E., Hus, V., Gan, W., Lu, F., Martin, D.M., Ousley, O., Guy, L., Bernier, R., Gerdts, J., Algermissen, M., Whitaker, A., Sutcliffe, J.S., Warren, Z., Klin, A., Saulnier, C., Hanson, E., Hundley, R., Piggot, J., Fombonne, E., Steiman, M., Miles, J., Kanne, S.M., Goin-Kochel, R.P., Peters, S.U., Cook, E.H., Guter, S., Tjernagel, J., Green-Snyder, L.A., Bishop, S., Esler, A., Gotham, K., Luyster, R., Miller, F., Olson, J., Richler, J., and Risi, S. (2012) A multisite study of the clinical diagnosis of different autism spectrum disorders. Archives of General Psychiatry **69**, 306–313.

Lord, C., Rutter, M., DiLavore, P.C., and Risi, S. (2002) Autism Diagnostic Observation Schedule, ADOS Manual. Los Angeles: Western Psychological Services.

Lord, C., Rutter, M., and Le Couteur, A. (1994) Autism Diagnostic Interview—Revised: a revised version of a diagnostic interview for caregivers of individuals with possible pervasive developmental disorders. Journal of Autism and Developmental Disorders **24**, 659–685.

Lounds Taylor, J., Dove, D., Veenstra-VanderWeele, J., Sathe, N.A., McPheeters, M.L., Jerome, R.N., and Warren, Z. (2012) Interventions for adolescents and young adults with autism spectrum disorders. Comparative effectiveness Review No. 65. (Prepared by the Venderbilt Evidence-based Practice Center under Contract No. 290-2007-10065-I.) AHRQ Publication no. 12-EHC063. In (Anonymous), Agency for Healthcare Research and Quality: Rockville, Maryland: Agency for Healthcare Research and Quality.

Malone, R. P., Gratz, S. S., Delaney, M. A., et al. (2005) Advances in drug treatments for children and adolescents with autism and other pervasive developmental disorders. CNS Drugs, **19**, 923–934.

McArthur, G.M. (2009) Auditory processing disorders: can they be treated? Current Opinion in Neurology. **22**, 137-43.

McDougle, C.J. (2016) Autism Spectrum Disorder. New York: Oxford University Press.

McDougle, C. J., Stigler, K. A. & Posey, D. J. (2003) Treatment of aggression in children and adolescents with autism and conduct disorder. Journal of Clinical Psychiatry, **64**, 16–25.

McNamee, R. (2003) Efficiency of two-phase designs for prevalence estimation. International Journal of Epidemiology **32**, 1072–1078.

Modabbernia, A., Velthorst, E., Reichenberg, A. (2017) Environmental risk factors for autism: an evidence-based review of systematic reviews and meta-analyses. Molecular Autism Brain, Cognition and Behaviour, **8**, 13. DOI: 10.1186/s13229-017-0121-4.

Narayanan, A. (2010) Effect of propranolol on functional connectivity in autism spectrum disorder: a pilot study.

National Institute for Health and Clinical Excellence (Great Britain) (2012) Autism: recognition, referral, diagnosis and management of adults on the autism spectrum. London: NICE.

Nylander, L. and Gillberg, C. (2001) Screening for autism spectrum disorders in adult psychiatric out-patients: a preliminary report. Acta Psychiatrica Scandinavica **103**, 428–434.

O'Nions, E., Tick, B., Rijsdijk, F., Happe, F., Plomin, R., Ronald, A., and Viding, E. (2015) Examining the genetic and environmental associations between autistic social and communication deficits and psychopathic callous-unemotional traits. PLoS One **10**, e0134331.

Parnas, J., Bovet, P., and Zahavi, D. (2002) Schizophrenic autism: clinical phenomenology and pathogenetic implications. World Psychiatry **1**, 131–136.

Perkins, E.A. (2016) Quality of life outcomes of aging adults and their families with autism and their families. In: Autism Spectrum Disorder in Mid and Later Life (ed. S. D. Wright), pp. 397–406. Philadelphia: Jessica Kingsley.

Pickles, A., Le, C.A., Leadbitter, K., Salomone, E., Cole-Fletcher, R., Tobin, H., Gammer, I., Lowry, J., Vamvakas, G., Byford, S., Aldred, C., Slonims, V., McConachie, H., Howlin, P., Parr, J.R., Charman, T., and Green, J. (2016) Parent-mediated social communication therapy for young children with autism (PACT): long-term follow-up of a randomised controlled trial. Lancet **388**, 2501–2509.

Popper, K. (1963) Conjectures and Refutations. London: Routledge & Kegan Paul.

Rai, D., Kerr, M.P., McManus, S., Jordanova, V., Lewis, G., and Brugha, T.S. (2012) Epilepsy and psychiatric comorbidity: a nationally representative population-based study. Epilepsia **53**, 1095–1103.

Ramos-Quiroga, J.A., Nasillo, V., Richarte, V., Corrales, M., Palma, F., Ibanez, P., Michelsen, M., Van de Glind, G., Casas, M., and Kooij, J.J. (2016) Criteria and concurrent validity of DIVA 2.0: a semi-structured diagnostic interview for adult ADHD. Journal of Attention Disorders Apr 28, pii: 1087054716646451. [Epub ahead of print]

Rapin, I. (2011) Autism turns 65: a neurologist's bird's eye view. In: Autism Spectrum Disorders (eds D. Amaral, G. Dawson, and D. H. Geschwind), pp. 3–16. New York: Oxford University Press.

Ritvo, R.A., Ritvo, E.R., Guthrie, D., Ritvo, M.J., Hufnagel, D.H., McMahon, W., Tonge, B., Mataix-Cols, D., Jassi, A., Attwood, T., and Eloff, J. (2011) The Ritvo Autism Asperger Diagnostic Scale-Revised (RAADS-R): a scale to assist the diagnosis of Autism Spectrum Disorder in adults: an international validation study. Journal of Autism and Developmental Disorders **41**, 1076–1089.

Robins, L.N. and Regier, D.A. (1991) Psychiatric Disorders in America: the Epidemiological Catchment Area Study. New York: Free Press (Macmillan Inc.).

Russell, A.J., Mataix-Cols, D., Anson, M., and Murphy, D.G. (2005) Obsessions and compulsions in Asperger syndrome and high-functioning autism. British Journal of Psychiatry **186**, 525–528.

Rydén, G., Rydén, E. and Hetta, J. (2008). Borderline personality disorder and autism spectrum disorder in females - a cross-sectional study. Clinical Neuropsychiatry **5**, 22-30.

Silberman, S. (2015) NeroTribes: the legacy of autism and how to think smarter about people who think differently. London: Allen & Unwin.

Skuse, D., Warrington, R., Bishop, D., Chowdhury, U., Lau, J., Mandy, W., and Place, M. (2004) The developmental, dimensional and diagnostic interview (3di): a novel computerized assessment for autism spectrum disorders. Journal of the American Academy of Child and Adolescent Psychiatry **43**, 548–558.

Sparrow, S.S., Balla, D.A., and Cicchetti, D.V. (1984) Vineland Adaptive Behavior Scales: Interview edition survey form. Circle Pines, MN: American Guidance Service.

Tantam, D. (2012) Autism Spectrum Disorder Throughout the Lifespan. London: Jessica Kingsley.

Turygin, N.C. and Matson, J.L. (2014) Adaptive behaviour, life skills, and leisure skills training for adolescents. In Adolescents and Adults with Autism Spectrum Disorders (eds F. R. Volkmar, R. Reichow, and J. C. McPartland), pp. 131–160. |New York: Springer.

Tyrer, F., Leaver, A., Lewis, S., Lovett, C., van Rensburg, K., Seaton, S., Smith, J., and Brugha, T. (2013) Testing adults for possible social and communication disorders, including autism spectrum disorders. Report to the National Institute for Health Research (NIHR) Collaboration for Leadership for Applied Health Research and Care (CLaHRC) for Leicestershire, Northamptonshire and Rutland (LLR)., p. 83. University of Leicester: Leicester.

Volkmar, F., Reichow, B., and McPartland, J.C. (2014) Adolescents and Adults with Autism Spectrum Disorders. New York: Springer.

Waterhouse, L., London, E., and Gillberg, C. (2016) ASD validity. Review Journal of Autism Developmental Disorders, **3**, 302–329.

White, T.P., Borgan, F., Ralley, O., and Shergill, S.S. (2016) You looking at me? Interpreting social cues in schizophrenia. Psychological Medicine **46**, 149–160.

Wing, J.K., Babor, T., Brugha, T., Burke, J., Cooper, J.E., Giel, R., Jablensky, A., Regier, D., and Sartorius, N. (1990) SCAN. Schedules for Clinical Assessment in Neuropsychiatry. Archives of General Psychiatry **47**, 589–593.

Wing, J.K., Cooper, J., and Sartorius, N. (1974) Measurement and Classification of Psychiatric Symptoms. Cambridge: Cambridge University Press.

Wing, L. (1981) Asperger's syndrome: a clinical account. Psychological Medicine **11**, 115–129.

Wing, L. (1993) The Diagnostic Interview for Social and Communication Disorders, 3rd edn. London: National Autistic Society.

Wing, L. (1997) The autistic spectrum. Lancet **350**, 1761–1766.

Wing, L. (2000) Diagnostic interview for social and communication disorders (DISCO) London: National Autistic Society.

Wing, L. and Gould, J. (1978) Systematic recording of behaviors and skills of retarded and psychotic children. Journal of Autism and Childhood Schizophrenia **8**, 79–97.

Wing, L. and Gould, J. (1979) Severe impairments of social interaction and associated abnormalities in children: epidemiology and classification. Journal of Autism and Developmental Disorders **9**, 11–29.

Wing, L., Leekam, S.R., Libby, S.J., Gould, J., and Larcombe, M. (2002) The Diagnostic Interview for Social and Communication Disorders: background, inter-rater reliability and clinical use. Journal of Child Psychology and Psychiatry **43**, 307–325.

Wing, L. and Shah, A. (2000) Catatonia in autistic spectrum disorders. British Journal of Psychiatry **176**, 357–362.

World Health Organization (1993) The ICD-10 Classification of Mental and Behavioural Disorders: diagnostic criteria for research. Geneva: WHO.

Wright, S.D. (2016) Autism Spectrum Disorder in Mid and Later Life. Philadelphia: Jessica Kingsley.

Wykes, T. and Sturt, E. (1986) The measurement of social behaviour in psychiatric patients: and assessment of the reliability and validity of the SBS schedule. British Journal of Psychiatry **148**, 1–11.

Index

Tables, figures, and boxes are indicated by an italic *t*, *f*, and *b* following the page number.

Aberrant Behavior Checklist (ABC) 173
abnormal psychological development 34–9
academic ability 175
active-but-odd 47
adaptive skills 188
Adult ADHD Self-Report Scale (ASRS) 102, 162
Adult Asperger Assessment (AAA) 114*t*, 115–16
adult autism
  alerting characteristics 16, 17–18*b*
  associated factors 10–12, 19*b*
  awareness of 13–31
  statutory guidance on support 9*b*
Adult Psychiatric Morbidity Surveys (APMS) 212, 225
alerting characteristics 16, 17–18*b*
alexithymia 51
aloofness 47
ambitendence 148*b*
anger 57, 58, 71
antidepressants 187, 190
antipsychotics 159, 187–8
anxiety 163–4
anxiolytic medication 159
app 199
appearance 149*b*
Applied Behaviour Analysis (ABA) 188
Asperger, H. 4, 5, 6
Asperger syndrome 5, 6–7
assessment
  advanced diagnostic 170–1
  carer initiation 66–7
  carer needs 205
  comorbidity 153–67
  developmental history 113–25, 158–60
  direct observation 137–52
  first impressions 97–9
  giving results to patients 183–4
  information 83–6
  initial (triage) 95–111
  interviewing patients 127–35
  multi-disciplinary approaches 174–5
  obtaining 79–94
  overview 77*f*
  patient needs 169–79
  population needs 213
  psychological 175–6
  reasoned case for 81–2
  specialist services 81
attention deficit hyperactivity disorder (ADHD) 97, 102, 162, 163, 175–6, 191
attention problems 175
atypical psychological development 34–9
audit 219
auditory processing disorder 191
auditory training 191
Australian Scale for Asperger Syndrome (ASAS) 88*t*
autism
  coining of term 5
  continuum 7
  definition 3–4
  history of 4–8
  spectrum concept 5
  under-recognition 157
Autism Act 2009 209–10, 211
Autism Behaviour Checklist (ABC) 91*t*, 173
Autism Diagnostic Interview (ADI) 115
Autism Diagnostic Interview, revised (ADI-R) 114*t*, 115, 170
Autism Diagnostic Observation Schedule (ADOS) 139–41, 170–1, 231, 235–6
AutisMe 199
Autism Programme Board for England 214
Autism Self-Assessment Framework (SAF) 212–13
Autism Spectrum Quotient (AQ) 89*t*, 92
Autism Spectrum Quotient-10 (AQ-10) 89*t*
automatic obedience 148*b*
awareness of adult autism 13–31

behaviour problems 58, 124–5
benefits system 202

binary decisions 14–15
bizarre behaviour 150*b*
bodily movements 51, 118, 123
body language 45–6, 121
borderline personality disorder 157, 166
brain abnormalities 38–9, 217
brain imaging 174
broader autism phenotype 11
bullying 48–9, 68

capacity 153–4, 192
care approaches 183–93
carers
　assessment initiation 66–7
　developmental assessment 113–16
　needs assessment 205
　questions for 105–6
　reasons for meeting 103–5
case vignettes 19–30
catatonia 147, 148–9*b*
central coherence 37
change, resistance to 55–8, 124
charities 204–5, 212, 213–14
chat rooms 62
chatting 44–5, 68–70, 120
childhood experience of autism 67–8
chilling out 70–1
chit chat 44–5, 68–70, 120
choice 197–8
circumscribed interests 57, 74, 131
clarity seeking 69
clinical course 158–60
Clinical Global Impression (CGI) 171, 173
clinical trials, status and outcome measures 171–4, 217–18
Clinton, Hillary 208
clothing 54, 72
clubs 204–5
cognitive ability 175
cognitive behaviour therapy (CBT) 190
cognitive difficulties, theories of 35–8
cognitive remediation 191
cognitive training 191
collections 56–7, 73–4
communication 17*b*
　childhood 119–21
　developmental differences 42–5
　infancy 42
　language 42–5, 119–21
　non-verbal 45–6, 98*t*, 103*t*, 121, 134, 142–4, 151*b*
　preferences 69–70
　social 102–3, 132–5, 146*b*, 146
　two-way 44–5, 68–70, 120

communication disorders 163
community interventions 188
comorbidity 10
　assessment 153–67
　treatment 189–91
　triage 96
computer analogy 64, 67
consent 84, 84*b*, 100*b*, 103, 192
conversation 44–5, 68–70, 120
co-ordination 58–9, 118
court proceedings 192, 204
creativity 122–3
criminal justice system 192, 204

danger awareness 150*b*
definition of autism 3–4
depression 156–7, 164
developmental coordination disorder (DCD) 163
developmental differences 39–59
Developmental, Dimensional and Diagnostic Interview (3di) 114*t*, 116
developmental history 113–25, 158–60
diagnosis 65, 71, 109
Diagnostic and Statistical Manual (DSM-IV) 42, 170
Diagnostic and Statistical Manual (DSM-5) 3, 6, 52, 107, 135, 147, 162, 163, 170
Diagnostic Interview for Social and Communication Disorders (DISCO) 41, 114*t*, 115, 116, 170
direct observation 34, 137–52
disability 66
distractibility 175
drug therapy 159, 187–8, 190

echopraxia 148*b*
education 118–19, 175, 193, 203
egocentrism 63
email 70
embarrassing behaviour 150*b*
emotional empathy 46
emotions, describing 51, 71–2
empathy 46
employment 65–6, 203
epidemiology 8–10, 157–8, 217, 225–6, 227–9
epilepsy 10, 58, 125, 166
EU
　Medicines Agency draft guidelines 191–2
　policy 210
executive functioning 37–8, 175

expert observation 34
explicit language 44
eye contact 49, 122, 151*b*
eye gaze 42, 49, 122, 142*b*, 143–4

facial expression 45, 121, 142*b*, 145, 151*b*
faith communities 204–5
family support 201
fascinations 55, 124
feelings
  describing ones own 51, 71–2
  of others 46
fine motor development 118
first impressions 97–9
flexibilitas cerea 148*b*
food preferences 54
forced grasping 148*b*
freezing 148*b*
friendship 48, 68, 70, 102, 122

GABA 39
gaze 42, 49, 122, 142*b*, 143–4
gender differences 10, 102–3, 145
general development 58, 59*b*
genetic counselling 189
genetic factors 11–12, 189
gesture 42, 45, 121, 141, 142*b*, 144, 151*b*
giggling 150*b*
Gilliam Autism Rating Scale (GARS/GARS-2) 88*t*
GPs 204
Grandin, Temple 73
grasping 148*b*
gross motor co-ordination 58–9, 118
group discussions 69
guided observation 34
gut microbiome 217

habits 73
Handicaps and Behaviour Schedule (MRC-HBC) 114*t*, 114–15
handshake 144
health care 150*b*
heritability 11–12, 189
hesitation 148*b*
history of autism 4–8
hoarding 31, 56–7, 150*b*
homeless 147, 204–5
housing 203
humour appreciation 43, 120

imagination 50–1, 122–3
imitation 39, 123
impact of symptoms 106–7

implicit language 44
inattention 175
independence 72–3, 119
infant development 42, 117–18
informants
  partners/peers 107–8
  questions for 105–6
  reasons for meeting 103–5
inheritance 11–12, 189
initial assessment (triage) 95–111
institutional settings 147, 149–50*b*
intellectual disability 160–2
interests 17–18*b*, 50–1, 73–4, 124, 150*b*
  circumscribed 57, 74, 131
International Classification of Diseases (ICD-10) 42, 85, 155, 166
International Classification of Diseases (ICD-11) 4, 155, 170
International Personality Disorder Examination (IPDE) 232
internet chat rooms 62
intervention, *see* treatment
interviews 34, 231–3
  direct patient interview 127–35
  informants, parents and carers 105–6
  questions for first meeting with patient 100–2
  self-expression problems 64
IQ 58

jerkiness 148*b*
joint referencing 42

Kanner, L. 4–5, 6

language 42–5, 119–21
laughter 150*b*
law 153–4, 192–3, 198–9, 204, 209–10, 211, 212
learning needs 218–19
legal issues 153–4, 192–3, 198–9, 204
legislation 199, 209–10, 211, 212
leisure facilities 204
literal understanding 43–4, 69, 119–20
long-term care settings 147, 149–50*b*

magnetic resonance imaging 174
make believe 50, 122–3
mannerisms 148*b*, 149*b*
masking symptoms 156–7
Medical Research Council Handicaps and Behaviour Schedule (MRC-HBC) 114*t*, 114–15
medications 159, 187–8, 190

meeting and greeting 97–9
melt downs 157
mental capacity 153–4, 192
mental health service 201–2
mental rigidity 55, 132, 155–6
mind blindness 37
mirror neurones 39
misaphonia 30–1
mortality 10
motor development 58–9, 118
movements 51, 118, 123
multi-disciplinary approaches 174–5

National Autistic Society 62
needs assessment
  carers 205
  patients 169–79
  population 213
negative posture 151*b*
negativism 148*b*
neural connectivity 38–9
neurobiology 38–9, 217
neurodiversity 7–8
neuroimaging 174
NICE guidelines 87, 92, 127, 160, 175, 186
non-verbal communication 45–6, 98*t*, 103*t*, 121, 134, 142–4, 151*b*

observation 34, 137–52
obsessions 55
obsessive compulsive disorder (OCD) 55, 156, 164
occupation 203
occupational therapy 177–8, 205
olfaction 54
online chat rooms 62
online communication 69–70
opposition 148*b*
outcome measures 171–4, 217–18
oversensitivity to sensory stimulation 53–4, 73, 124
oxytocin 217

pain sensitivity 54
parents
  questions for 105–6
  reasons for meeting 103–5
  support for 201
  see also carers
partners as informants 107–8
passivity 47, 122
Past and Present Behaviour Schedule (PPBS) 113, 114*t*, 115, 116, 124

peers
  as informants 107–8
  relationships with 47, 68, 106, 122, 164
personal choice 197–8
personal hygiene 150*b*
personality disorder 157, 166
personalized budgets 201–2
personal passport 198, 199
perspective taking 63
pharmacotherapy 159, 187–8, 190
phenomenological approach 33–4
planning 50, 56, 71–2
play behaviour 50, 122–3
policy
  development 207–10
  effectiveness 212–13
  implementation 210–11, 213–14
politeness 65
population needs assessment 213
posturing 149*b*
predictability 73–4
pretence 50, 122–3
primary care 80, 81, 87, 92, 170, 171, 177, 200*b*
processing speed 175
professional peer groups 219
proximal sensory stimulation 52–3, 123
psychiatrists
  competencies 219*t*
  legal responsibilities 153, 192–3
  training 215–16
psychological assessment 175–6
psychological development
  theories 34–9
psychosis 34, 154, 165
psychosocial interventions 188, 202
psychotherapy 190–1
public health surveillance 213, 226
public misunderstanding 71

quality of life 178

rainbow metaphor 15
reasonable adjustments 153–4, 192, 198–9, 204
reciprocity 48
recreation facilities 204
referral
  alternatives to 82–3
  effective 81–2
  experiences and expectations 93–4
  information 83–6
  service choice 92–3
  test evaluation and use 86–92

relationships 133, 135
  breakdowns 67
  friendship 48, 68, 70, 102, 122
  peers 47, 68, 106, 122, 164
repetitive behaviours 52–3, 55–8, 73–4, 123, 130–2, 156
repetitive transcranial magnetic stimulation (rTMS) 191
Research Autism 186–7
research design 35
researcher bias 35
research priorities 216–18
resistance to change 55–8, 124
restriction of liberty 153–4
rigidity 55, 132, 155–6
risk assessment and management 125, 153, 160–1, 175, 192–3, 202
risk behaviour 10, 23, 25, 26, 58, 85, 94, 104*b*, 105, 125, 160, 165, 174, 176, 185, 192
rituals 57–8, 73, 131
Ritvo Autism Asperger Diagnostic Scale Revised (RAADS-R) 90*t*, 92
Ritvo–Freeman Real-life Rating Scale (RF–RLRS) 171–3
routines 55–8, 124, 131
rumination 155–6

safeguarding 200
Sally Ann Test 36
sameness 73–4
SCAN interview 127, 156, 232, 233
schizoid personality disorder 166
schizophrenia 142, 165
school work 118–19, 175
self-care 118
self-diagnosis 83
self-expression 64
self-harm 10, 123, 125, 150*b*, 160–1
self-identity 164
self-neglect 125, 150*b*
self-reports 92, 115, 162
self-stimulation 52–3
sensory differences 51–4, 73, 123, 132
sensory stimulation, sensitivity to 53–4, 73, 124
serotonin 39
services
  mental health 201–2
  referral choice 92–3
  specialist 81
service sector industry 212
sex differences 10, 102–3, 145
shaking hands 144

sharing of interest 42
siblings 74, 120–1
smartphone app 199
smell 54
Social and Communication Disorders Checklist (SCDC) 91*t*
social anxiety disorder 164
social awareness 121
social care 195–205
  effectiveness 196–7
  personal choice 197–8
social communication 102–3, 132–5, 146*b*, 146
Social Communication Questionnaire (SCQ) 89*t*
social curiosity 134
social functioning 70–1
social interactions 17*b*, 46–9, 102, 121–2, 132–5, 143*b*
social intuition 134
social passivity 47, 122
social phobia 164
social (pragmatic) communication disorder 162–3
Social Responsiveness Scale (SRS) 89*t*, 173
social skills training 189
social work 176–7, 199–200, 201–2
sociopathy 166
sound sensitivity 53–4, 124
specialist services 81
spectrum concept 5
speech and language therapy 176
staring 49
status measures 171–4
stereotypies 51, 149*b*
study design 35
substantia nigra 55
subthreshold symptoms 14
suicidality 10, 28, 125, 158, 165
supported employment 203
surveillance 213, 226
symptoms
  impact of 106–7
  masking and amplification 156–7
  subthreshold 14

taste 54, 73
temperature sensitivity 54
text messages 69
texture 54
theory of mind 36–7
third sector organizations 212, 213–14
tone of voice 45, 120, 142*b*, 145, 151*b*

training
  auditory 191
  cognitive 191
  employment 65–6
  psychiatrists 215–16
  social skills 189
  workforce retraining 211–12
transcranial magnetic stimulation (rTMS) 191
treatment 183–93
  adaptive skills 188
  community interventions 188
  comorbidities 189–91
  EU Medicines Agency draft guidelines 191–2
  goals and targets 184–5
  guidelines and evidence of effectiveness 185–6
  outcome measures used in studies 171–4
  pharmacotherapy 159, 187–8, 190
  psychosocial 188, 202
  psychotherapy 190–1
  response 159
  social skills training 189
triage 95–111
two-way interaction 44–5, 68–70, 120

UK policy 208, 209–10
under-recognition of autism 157
US
  policy 208–9
  surveillance 213, 226

Vineland Adaptive Behavior Scales (VABS), Maladaptive Sub-scale 173
visual stimuli, response to 54, 124
visuospatial skills 118
vocal intonation 45, 120, 142*b*, 145, 151*b*
vulnerability 200

welfare benefits 202
Wing, L. 5, 39, 50, 55
workforce retraining 211–12
work settings 65–6, 203
World Health Organization Schedules for Clinical Assessment in Neuropsychiatry (WHO SCAN) 127, 156, 232, 233
worry 155–6

Yale–Brown Obsessive Compulsive Scale (YBOCS) 171, 173